W9-BKZ-317

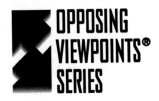
OPPOSING
VIEWPOINTS®
SERIES

Genetic Engineering

Other Books of Related Interest:

Opposing Viewpoints Series

Genetic Disorders

At Issue Series

Genetically Modified Food

Are Adult Stem Cells as Valuable as Embryonic Stem Cells?

The Ethics of Cloning

"Congress shall make no law. . .abridging the freedom of speech, or of the press."

First Amendment to the U.S. Constitution

The basic foundation of our democracy is the First Amendment guarantee of freedom of expression. The *Opposing Viewpoints* Series is dedicated to the concept of this basic freedom and the idea that it is more important to practice it than to enshrine it.

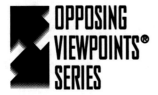

OPPOSING VIEWPOINTS® SERIES

Genetic Engineering

David M. Haugen and Susan Musser, Book Editors

GREENHAVEN PRESS
A part of Gale, Cengage Learning

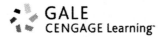

GALE
CENGAGE Learning™

Detroit • New York • San Francisco • New Haven, Conn • Waterville, Maine • London

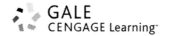

Christine Nasso, *Publisher*
Elizabeth Des Chenes, *Managing Editor*

© 2009 Greenhaven Press, a part of Gale, Cengage Learning

Gale and Greenhaven Press are registered trademarks used herein under license.

For more information, contact:
Greenhaven Press
27500 Drake Rd.
Farmington Hills, MI 48331-3535
Or you can visit our Internet site at gale.cengage.com

For product information and technology assistance, contact us at

Gale Customer Support, 1-800-877-4253
For permission to use material from this text or product, submit all requests online at www.cengage.com/permissions

Further permissions questions can be emailed to permissionrequest@cengage.com

Articles in Greenhaven Press anthologies are often edited for length to meet page requirements. In addition, original titles of these works are changed to clearly present the main thesis and to explicitly indicate the author's opinion. Every effort is made to ensure that Greenhaven Press accurately reflects the original intent of the authors. Every effort has been made to trace the owners of copyrighted material.

Cover image copyright Andrea Danti, 2008. Used under license from Shutterstock.com.

LIBRARY OF CONGRESS CATALOGING-IN-PUBLICATION DATA

Genetic engineering / David M. Haugen and Susan Musser, book editors.
    p. cm. -- (Opposing viewpoints)
Includes bibliographical references and index.
ISBN 978-0-7377-4368-5 (hardcover)
ISBN 978-0-7377-4367-8 (pbk.)
1. Genetic engineering. 2. Genetic engineering--Social aspects. I. Haugen, David M., 1969- II. Musser, Susan.
QH442.G446 2009
174'.957--dc22
                                                          2008035440

Printed in the United States of America
2 3 4 5 6   13 12 11 10 09

ED271

Chapter 4: How Should Genetic Engineering Technology Be Regulated?

Why Consider
Opposing Viewpoints?

> *"The only way in which a human being can make some approach to knowing the whole of a subject is by hearing what can be said about it by persons of every variety of opinion and studying all modes in which it can be looked at by every character of mind. No wise man ever acquired his wisdom in any mode but this."*
>
> *John Stuart Mill*

In our media-intensive culture it is not difficult to find differing opinions. Thousands of newspapers and magazines and dozens of radio and television talk shows resound with differing points of view. The difficulty lies in deciding which opinion to agree with and which "experts" seem the most credible. The more inundated we become with differing opinions and claims, the more essential it is to hone critical reading and thinking skills to evaluate these ideas. Opposing Viewpoints books address this problem directly by presenting stimulating debates that can be used to enhance and teach these skills. The varied opinions contained in each book examine many different aspects of a single issue. While examining these conveniently edited opposing views, readers can develop critical thinking skills such as the ability to compare and contrast authors' credibility, facts, argumentation styles, use of persuasive techniques, and other stylistic tools. In short, the Opposing Viewpoints Series is an ideal way to attain the higher-level thinking and reading skills so essential in a culture of diverse and contradictory opinions.

In addition to providing a tool for critical thinking, Opposing Viewpoints books challenge readers to question their own strongly held opinions and assumptions. Most people form their opinions on the basis of upbringing, peer pressure, and personal, cultural, or professional bias. By reading carefully balanced opposing views, readers must directly confront new ideas as well as the opinions of those with whom they disagree. This is not to simplistically argue that everyone who reads opposing views will—or should—change his or her opinion. Instead, the series enhances readers' understanding of their own views by encouraging confrontation with opposing ideas. Careful examination of others' views can lead to the readers' understanding of the logical inconsistencies in their own opinions, perspective on why they hold an opinion, and the consideration of the possibility that their opinion requires further evaluation.

Evaluating Other Opinions

To ensure that this type of examination occurs, Opposing Viewpoints books present all types of opinions. Prominent spokespeople on different sides of each issue as well as well-known professionals from many disciplines challenge the reader. An additional goal of the series is to provide a forum for other, less known, or even unpopular viewpoints. The opinion of an ordinary person who has had to make the decision to cut off life support from a terminally ill relative, for example, may be just as valuable and provide just as much insight as a medical ethicist's professional opinion. The editors have two additional purposes in including these less known views. One, the editors encourage readers to respect others' opinions—even when not enhanced by professional credibility. It is only by reading or listening to and objectively evaluating others' ideas that one can determine whether they are worthy of consideration. Two, the inclusion of such viewpoints encourages the important critical thinking skill of objectively evaluating an author's credentials and bias. This evaluation will illuminate an author's reasons for taking a particular stance on an issue and will aid in readers' evaluation of the author's ideas.

It is our hope that these books will give readers a deeper understanding of the issues debated and an appreciation of the complexity of even seemingly simple issues when good and honest people disagree. This awareness is particularly important in a democratic society such as ours in which people enter into public debate to determine the common good. Those with whom one disagrees should not be regarded as enemies but rather as people whose views deserve careful examination and may shed light on one's own.

Thomas Jefferson once said that "difference of opinion leads to inquiry, and inquiry to truth." Jefferson, a broadly educated man, argued that "if a nation expects to be ignorant and free . . . it expects what never was and never will be." As individuals and as a nation, it is imperative that we consider the opinions of others and examine them with skill and discernment. The Opposing Viewpoints Series is intended to help readers achieve this goal.

David L. Bender and Bruno Leone,
Founders

Introduction

> "New technologies of the Genetic Age allow scientists, corporations and governments to manipulate the natural world at the most fundamental level—the genetic one. Imagine the wholesale transfer of genes between totally unrelated species and across all biological boundaries—plant, animal and human—creating thousands of novel life forms in a brief moment of evolutionary time. Then, with clonal propagation, mass-producing countless replicas of these new creations, releasing them into the biosphere to propagate, mutate, proliferate and migrate. This is, in fact, the radical scientific and commercial experiment now underway." —Jeremy Rifkin, "The Biotech Century," emagazine.com, May/June 1998.

Genetic engineering is the alteration of an organism through manipulation of its genetic structure. The alteration can be across different species or within a single species, and any genetic trait that is changed may be passed down to the progeny of the altered organisms. Genetic engineering typically involves splicing deoxyribonucleic acid (DNA) or DNA fragments and inserting the spliced segment into a host organism. In 2003, for example, pet stores began marketing zebrafish that had a jellyfish gene inserted into them that allowed them to glow in the dark. Similarly, scientists have engineered tomatoes that possess a flounder gene which allows the vegetables to resist cold temperatures in the same manner the fish tolerates cold waters. In more unusual cases, entire organisms have been cloned by transferring a nucleus from a living organism into an egg that lacks a nucleus. The famed sheep, Dolly, was "born" in this manner from the nucleus of a mammary cell of an adult ewe. In all these instances, genetic material was removed from a donor and inserted into a host, producing a novel organism that did not come about through traditional breeding.

The novelty of genetic engineering is behind much of the controversy over its use. Except for horticultural cloning, which has been practiced for thousands of years, most forms of genetic manipulation are products of the late twentieth century. Gene splicing technology of the 1970s and 1980s, the cloning of Dolly in 1996, and the release of a complete map of the human genome in 2003 illustrate that genetic engineering has made great strides in a short period of time. And as with most sciences still in their infancies, genetic engineering cannot claim that its practices are perfected; any long term consequences of its use are still a matter of speculation. In addition, the failures of many genetic experiments fuel the fears people have about its implementation. For example, though Dolly the sheep was a successful product of cloning, her life was cut short by lung cancer, leaving a lasting—if erroneous—impression that her disease and death were the results of her unnatural birth. More distressing, however, are those instances in which dangers *are* directly attributable to genetic modification. In 1993, certain commercial-grade soybeans were injected with a gene from a Brazil nut to increase their protein levels. Unfortunately, the soybeans caused immunological reactions in people who had nut allergies, forcing the manufacturer to cease production and dispose of the test products.

These incidents contribute to the divisive opinions Americans have about genetic engineering. A 2006 Pew Initiative poll revealed that 34 percent of Americans believe genetically modified (GM) foods are safe to eat while 29 percent contend that they are unsafe. The same poll showed that 61 percent of Americans are uncomfortable with animal cloning. Other polls indicate that more than 80 percent of Americans oppose human reproductive cloning, and roughly 60 percent oppose the use of embryonic cloning techniques to aid cures for human diseases. Many of those polled are afraid of what could go wrong with such new technology; others simply find practices such as cloning immoral. The environmental organization Friends of the Earth warns that genetic engineering could "propel us into a 'brave new world'" in which human beings' relationships with the earth and each other are ethically compromised. If genetic engineering is not halted, predicts the group, it will result in a dystopia that will succeed in only "devaluing each individual and completing the divorce from nature that began a long time ago."

Not everyone, though, fears a genetically engineered future. Some see genetic engineering as an acceleration of a natural evolutionary process that otherwise might take thousands of years to unfold. After all, cloning takes place in the natural world, and crossbreeding is certainly not a new phenomenon. From advances in genetic engineering, advocates claim that livestock can be made to produce leaner meat and food crops can be made resistant to disease and pests. Even "unnatural" alterations, such as the use of gene therapy to treat human diseases, could be beneficial if they deliver on their promise. As the Nemours Foundation, a children's health organization, proclaimed, "With its potential to eliminate and prevent hereditary diseases such as cystic fibrosis and hemophilia and its use as a possible cure for heart disease, AIDS, and cancer, gene therapy is a potential medical miracleworker." Furthermore, the more radical notion of genetically enhancing human traits—such as height, intelligence, and talent—even has its supporters in the transhumanist movement. Transhumanists believe in expanding human development by any means to reach other, higher modes of being. As Oxford University scholar and transhumanist philosopher Nick Bostrom avers, "Transhumanism promotes the quest to develop further so that we can explore hitherto inaccessible realms of value. Technological enhancement of human organisms is a means that we ought to pursue to this end."

With supporters and detractors and their equally compelling visions of genetically engineered utopias and dystopias, the future of genetic engineering is still a subject of hot debate in America. State legislatures have addressed bills concerning the production of GM crops, while Congress has in recent years seen the introduction and reintroduction of the Human Cloning Prohibition Act—a bill that has yet to garner enough support to pass. Those lawmakers and interest groups that are concerned over the dangers of genetic engineering insist that legal action cannot come soon enough. In pushing for a California bill that would hold GM crop manufacturers liable for contamination of traditional crops, Rebecca Spector of the Center for Food Safety claimed, "Farmers nationally have suffered economic losses from unintentional contamination of their crops with (genetically engineered) materials." Similarly, Senator Mary Landrieu of Louisiana, a cosponsor of the Human Cloning Prohibition Act, maintains that "we need only to turn on the evening news to see that human cloning is a very real and present concern." The sense of urgency is palpable in their warnings, making the topic a national controversy that has commanded the attention of government, the media, and the public.

In this anthology, *Opposing Viewpoints: Genetic Engineering*, several lawmakers, journalists, scientists, and policy advocates debate the practice of genetic engineering and capture much of the urgency surrounding the issue. In chapters titled Should Genetic Engineering on Humans Be Permitted? Is Genetic Engineering Ethical? What Is the Impact of Genetically Engineered Foods? and How Should Genetic Engineering

Technology Be Regulated? these commentators examine the environmental, social, and moral impact of genetic engineering on the nation and the world. They not only offer predictions of what may come of the widespread use of genetic engineering but also address the current effects of this technology and the ways in which it has already shaped how people think about food, reproduction, consumerism, identity, and what it means to be human in the brave new world.

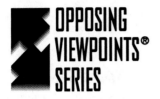

OPPOSING
VIEWPOINTS®
SERIES

 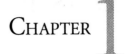

Should Genetic Engineering on Humans Be Permitted?

Chapter Preface

In June 2008, the *New England Journal of Medicine* reported that researchers had successfully used immunotherapy to counter an advanced stage of melanoma in a fifty-two-year-old man. The doctors had removed CD4+ T cells, a type of white blood cell arising from stem cells found in the patient's bone marrow; these cells, "were then expanded vastly in the laboratory using modifications to existing methods [of cloning]." After modification, around five billion of these cloned cells were infused back into the patient. After two months, tests showed the man to be free from cancerous tumors, and two years later, his melanoma has continued to remain in remission.

Cassian Yee, an associate member of the Clinical Research Division at Fred Hutchinson Cancer Research Center and the leader of the research team responsible for the study, reported that his team "was surprised by the anti-tumor effect of these CD4 T cells and its duration of response." Yee noted, "For this patient we were successful, but we would need to confirm the effectiveness of therapy in a larger study." He also cautioned that this therapy worked for this specific patient's immune system because the patient's tumor cells expressed a certain antigen. Yee stated that the treatment may not be consistent for all cases of late-stage melanoma. He also predicted that this therapy would work in 25 percent of cases where the patient has the same immune system type and same tumor antigens.

The cloned cells that were infused into the patient were antigen specific to the antigen NY-ESO-1 found in the patient's tumor cells. Although only 50 to 75 percent of the tumor cells contained this antigen, after the infusion the entire tumor shrank in response. Yee's results are a major breakthrough in immunotherapy. This growing field of medical research uses the patient's immune system—in this case, adult stem cells—to fight cancer in an attempt to reduce the need for highly toxic treatments, such as chemotherapy and radiation.

The use of adult stem cells in medical therapies has been a growing trend since the discovery that they could successfully treat leukemia, as well as be used to grow new blood vessels and heart muscle in patients. These breakthroughs also demonstrated that adult stem cells could be used as an alternative to the more controversial embryonic stem cells in medical research and testing.

In the following chapter, President George W. Bush praises the use of adult stem cells as viable therapeutic tools in remedying human diseases and disorders. President Bush believes that the work of Yee and others proves that genetic engineering on humans can be performed safely and need not involve the harvesting of embryonic cells, which, in his view, sacrifices nascent human life. Other authors in the chapter discuss whether tampering with the human genome will always yield benefits that outweigh the risks of such experimentation.

> *"Every day that the introduction of effective human genetic enhancement is delayed is a day of lost individual and cultural potential."*

Human Genetic Engineering Will Prove Beneficial and Should Be Allowed

Nick Bostrom

In the following viewpoint, Nick Bostrom champions genetic enhancement as a means to make people smarter, healthier, and more talented. He argues against claims that genetic engineering would lead to a dystopian future in which those who could afford enhancements would live superior lives to those who could not. Instead, he maintains, society could easily build in safeguards that would promote social justice in the use of genetic engineering. Nick Bostrom is a philosopher at Oxford University in England and the director of the Oxford Future of Humanity Institute. He is an advocate of transhumanism, a philosophical movement that seeks to improve human life and society through any means, including cloning and genetic enhancement.

Nick Bostrom, "Human Genetic Enhancements: A Transhumanist Perspective," *Journal of Value Inquiry*, vol. 37, no. 4, December 7, 2003, pp. 493–506. Reproduced with kind permission from Springer Science and Business Media, conveyed through Copyright Clearance Center, Inc., and the author.

As you read, consider the following questions:

1. Why does Bostrom believe that critics of genetic engineering are actually valuable to the cause of advancing human genetic enhancement?

2. As the author describes them, what are "externalities" and how are they applied to his view of genetic enhancement?

3. What does Bostrom say are some of the ways in which the "inequality-increasing tendencies" of enhancement technologies might be counteracted by social policies?

Transhumanism is a loosely defined movement that has developed gradually over the past two decades. It promotes an interdisciplinary approach to understanding and evaluating the opportunities for enhancing the human condition and the human organism opened up by the advancement of technology. Attention is given to both present technologies, like genetic engineering and information technology, and anticipated future ones, such as molecular nanotechnology and artificial intelligence. . . .

Transhumanists view human nature as a work-in-progress, a half-baked beginning that we can learn to remold in desirable ways. Current humanity need not be the endpoint of evolution. Transhumanists hope that by responsible use of science, technology, and other rational means we shall eventually manage to become post-human, beings with vastly greater capacities than present human beings have. . . .

Transhumanism promotes the quest to develop further so that we can explore hitherto inaccessible realms of value. Technological enhancement of human organisms is a means that we ought to pursue to this end. . . .

Most potential human enhancement technologies have so far received scant attention in the ethics literature. One exception is genetic engineering, the morality of which has been extensively debated in recent years. To illustrate how the transhumanist approach can be applied to particular technologies, we shall therefore ... turn to consider the case of human germ-line genetic enhancements.

Certain types of objection against germ-line modifications are not accorded much weight by a transhumanist interlocutor. For instance, objections that are based on the idea that there is something inherently wrong or morally suspect in using science to manipulate human nature are regarded by transhumanists as wrongheaded. Moreover, transhumanists emphasize that particular concerns about negative aspects of genetic enhancements, even when such concerns are legitimate, must be judged against the potentially enormous benefits that could come from genetic technology successfully employed. For example, many commentators worry about the psychological effects of the use of germ-line engineering. The ability to select the genes of our children and to create so-called designer babies will, it is claimed, corrupt parents, who will come to view their children as mere products. We will then begin to evaluate our offspring according to standards of quality control, and this will undermine the ethical ideal of unconditional acceptance of children, no matter what their abilities and traits. Are we really prepared to sacrifice on the altar of consumerism even those deep values that are embodied in traditional relationships between child and parents? Is the quest for perfection worth this cultural and moral cost? A transhumanist should not dismiss such concerns as irrelevant. Transhumanists recognize that the depicted outcome would be bad. We do not want parents to love and respect their children less. We do not want social prejudice against people with disabilities to get worse. The psychological and cultural effects of commodifying human nature are potentially important.

But such dystopian scenarios are speculations. There is no firm ground for believing that the alleged consequences would actually happen. What relevant evidence we have, for instance regarding the treatment of children who have been conceived through the use of in vitro fertilization or embryo screening, suggests that the pessimistic prognosis is alarmist. Parents will in fact love and respect their children even when artificial means and conscious choice play a part in procreation.

We might speculate, instead, that germ-line enhancements will lead to more love and parental dedication. Some mothers and fathers might find it easier to love a child who, thanks to enhancements, is bright, beautiful, healthy, and happy. The practice of germ-line enhancement might lead to better treatment of people with disabilities, because a general demystification of the genetic contributions to human traits could make it clearer that people with disabilities are not to blame for their disabilities and a decreased incidence of some disabilities could lead to more assistance being available for the remaining affected people to enable them to live full, unrestricted lives through various technological and social supports. Speculating about possible psychological or cultural effects of germ-line engineering can therefore cut both ways. Good consequences no less than bad ones are possible. In the absence of sound arguments for the view that the negative consequences would predominate, such speculations provide no reason against moving forward with the technology.

Ruminations over hypothetical side-effects may serve to make us aware of things that could go wrong so that we can be on the lookout for untoward developments. By being aware of the perils in advance, we will be in a better position to take preventive countermeasures. . . . To the extent that the critics have done their job, they can alert us to many of the potential untoward consequences of germ-line engineering and contribute to our ability to take precautions, thus improving the odds that the balance of effects will be positive. There may well be some negative consequences of human germ-line engineering that we will not forestall, though of course the mere existence of negative effects is not a decisive reason not to proceed. Every major technology has some negative consequences. Only

An Idyllic Vision of the Future

By 2100 the typical American may attend a family reunion in which five generations are playing together. The great-great-great-grandma is 150 years old, and she will be as vital as she was when she was 30 and as vital as her 30-year-old great-great-grandson, with whom she's playing touch football. After the game, she'll enjoy a plate of salad greens filled with not only a full day's worth of nutrients but the medicines she needs to repair the damage to her aging cells. She'll be able to chat about the academic discipline—maybe economics—that she studied in the 1980s with as much acuity and depth of knowledge and memory as her 50-year-old great-granddaughter who is now studying the same thing.

Ronald Bailey, Reason, *January 2006.*

after a fair comparison of the risks with the likely positive consequences can any conclusion based on a cost-benefit analysis be reached.

In the case of germ-line enhancements, the potential gains are enormous. Only rarely, however, are the potential gains discussed, perhaps because they are too obvious to be of much theoretical interest. By contrast, uncovering subtle and nontrivial ways in which manipulating our genome could undermine deep values is philosophically a lot more challenging. But if we think about it, we recognize that the promise of genetic enhancements is anything but insignificant. Being free from severe genetic diseases would be good, as would having a mind that can learn more quickly, or having a more robust immune system. Healthier, wittier, happier people may be able to reach new levels culturally. To achieve a significant enhancement of human capacities would be to embark on the transhuman journey of exploration of some of the modes of being that are not accessible to us as we are currently constituted, possibly to discover and to instantiate important new values. On an even more basic level, genetic engineering holds great potential for alleviating unnecessary human suffering. Every day that the introduction of effective human genetic enhancement is delayed is a day of lost individual and cultural potential, and a day of torment for many unfortunate sufferers of diseases that could have been prevented. Seen in this light, proponents of a ban or a moratorium on human genetic modification must take on a heavy burden of proof in order to have the balance of reason tilt in their favor. Transhumanists conclude that the challenge has not been met.

Should Human Reproduction Be Regulated?

One way of going forward with genetic engineering is to permit everything, leaving all choices to parents. While this attitude may be consistent with transhumanism, it is not the best transhumanist approach. One thing that can be said for adopting a libertarian stance in regard to human reproduction is the sorry track record of socially planned attempts to improve the human gene pool. The list of historical examples of state intervention in this domain ranges from the genocidal horrors of the Nazi regime, to the incomparably milder but still disgraceful semi-coercive sterilization programs of mentally impaired individuals favored by many well-meaning socialists in the past century, to the controversial but perhaps understandable program of the current Chinese government to limit population growth. In each case, state policies interfered with the reproductive choices of individuals. If parents had been left to make the choices for themselves, the worst transgressions of the eugenics movement would not have occurred. Bearing this in mind, we ought to think twice before giving our support to any proposal that would have the state regulate what sort of children people are allowed to have and the methods that may be used to conceive them.

We currently permit governments to have a role in reproduction and child-rearing and we may reason by extension that there would likewise be a role in regulating the application of genetic reproductive technology. State agencies and regulators play a supportive and supervisory role, attempting to promote the interests of the child. Courts intervene in cases of child abuse or neglect. Some social policies are in place to support children from disadvantaged backgrounds and to ameliorate some of the worst inequities suffered by children from poor homes, such as through the provision of free schooling. These measures have analogues that apply to genetic enhancement technologies. For example, we ought to outlaw genetic modifications that are intended to damage the child or limit its opportunities in life, or that are judged to be too risky. If there are basic enhancements that would be beneficial for a child but that some parents cannot afford, then we should consider subsidizing those enhancements, just as we do with basic education. . . .

Externalities

An externality, as understood by economists, is a cost or a benefit of an action that is not carried by a decision-maker. An example of a negative externality might be found in a firm that lowers its production costs by polluting the environment. The firm enjoys most of the benefits while escaping the costs, such as environmental degradation, which may instead be paid by people living nearby. Externalities can also be positive, as when people put time and effort into creating a beautiful garden outside their house. The effects are enjoyed not exclusively by the gardeners but spill over to passersby. As a rule of thumb, sound social policy and social norms would have us internalize many externalities so that the incentives of producers more closely match the social value of production. We may levy a pollution tax on the polluting firm, for instance, and give our praise to the home gardeners who beautify the neighborhood.

Genetic enhancements aimed at the obtainment of goods that are desirable only in so far as they provide a competitive advantage tend to have negative externalities. An example of such a positional good, as economists call them, is stature. There is evidence that being tall is statistically advantageous, at least for men in Western societies. Taller men earn more money, wield greater social influence, and are viewed as more sexually attractive. Parents wanting to give their child the best possible start in life may rationally choose a genetic enhancement that adds an inch or two to the expected length of their offspring. Yet for society as a whole, there seems to be no advantage whatsoever in people being taller. If everybody grew two inches, nobody would be better off than they were before. Money spent on a positional good like length has little or no net effect on social welfare and is therefore, from society's point of view, wasted.

Health is a very different type of good. It has intrinsic benefits. If we become healthier, we are personally better off and others are not any worse off. There may even be a positive externality of enhancing our own health. If we are less likely to contract a contagious disease, others benefit by being less likely to get infected by us. Being healthier, you may also contribute more to society and consume less of publicly funded healthcare.

If we were living in a simple world where people were perfectly rational self-interested economic agents and where social policies had no costs or unintended effects, then the basic policy prescription regarding genetic enhancements would be relatively straightforward. We should internalize the externalities of genetic enhancements by taxing enhancements that have negative externalities and subsidizing enhancements that have positive externalities. Unfortunately, crafting policies that work well in practice is considerably more difficult. Even determining the net size of the externalities of a particular genetic enhancement can be difficult. There is clearly an intrinsic value to enhancing memory or intelligence in as much as most of us would like to be a bit smarter, even if that did not have the slightest effect on our standing in relation to others. But there would also be important externalities, both positive and negative. On the negative side, others would suffer some disadvantage from our increased brainpower in that their own competitive situation would be worsened. Being more intelligent, we would be more likely to attain high-status positions in society, positions that would otherwise have been enjoyed by a competitor. On the positive side, others might benefit from enjoying witty conversations with us and from our increased taxes.

If in the case of intelligence enhancement the positive externalities outweigh the negative ones, then a prima facie case exists not only for permitting genetic enhancements aimed at increasing intellectual ability, but for encouraging and subsidizing them too. Whether such policies remain a good idea when all practicalities of implementation and political realities are taken into account is another matter. But at least we can conclude that an enhancement that has both significant intrinsic benefits for an enhanced individual and net positive externalities for the rest of society should be encouraged. By contrast, enhancements that confer only positional advantages, such as augmentation of stature or physical attractiveness, should not be socially encouraged, and we might even attempt to make a case for social policies aimed at reducing expenditure on such goods, for instance through a progressive tax on consumption.

The Issue of Equality

One important kind of externality in germ-line enhancements is their effects on social equality. This has been a focus for many opponents of germ-line genetic engineering who worry that it will widen the gap between haves and have-nots. Today, children from wealthy homes enjoy many environmental privileges, including access to better schools and social networks. Arguably, this constitutes an inequity against children from poor homes. We can imagine scenarios where such inequities grow much larger thanks to genetic interventions that only the rich can afford, adding genetic advantages to the environmental advantages already benefiting privileged children. We could even speculate about the members of the privileged stratum of society eventually enhancing themselves and their offspring to a point where the human species, for many practical purposes, splits into two or more species that have little in common except a shared evolutionary history. The genetically privileged might become ageless, healthy, super-geniuses of flawless physical beauty, who are graced with a sparkling wit and a disarmingly self-deprecating sense of humor, radiating warmth, empathetic charm, and relaxed confidence. The non-privileged would remain as people are today but perhaps deprived of some their self-respect and suffering occasional bouts of envy. The mobility between the lower and the upper classes might disappear, and a child born to poor parents, lacking genetic enhancements, might find it impossible to successfully compete against the super-children of the rich. Even if no discrimination or exploitation of the lower class occurred, there is still something disturbing about the prospect of a society with such extreme inequalities.

While we have vast inequalities today and regard many of these as unfair, we also accept a wide range of inequalities because we think that they are deserved, have social benefits, or are unavoidable concomitants to free individuals making their own and sometimes foolish choices about how to live their lives. Some of these justifications can also be used to exonerate some inequalities that could result from germ-line engineering. Moreover, the increase in unjust inequalities due to technology is not a sufficient reason for discouraging the development and use of the technology. We must also consider its benefits, which include not only positive externalities but also intrinsic values that reside in such goods as the enjoyment of health, a soaring mind, and emotional well-being.

We can also try to counteract some of the inequality-increasing tendencies of enhancement technology with social policies. One way of doing so would be by widening access to the technology by subsidizing it or providing it for free to children of poor parents. In cases where the enhancement has considerable positive externalities, such a policy may actually benefit everybody, not just the recipients of the subsidy. In other cases, we could support the policy on the basis of social justice and solidarity. . . .

All of this is based on the hypothesis that germ-line engineering would in fact increase inequalities if left unregulated and no countermeasures were taken. That hypothesis might be false. In particular, it might turn out to be technologically easier to cure gross genetic defects than to enhance an already healthy genetic constitution. We currently know much more about many specific inheritable diseases, some of which are due to single gene defects, than we do about the genetic basis of talents and desirable qualities such as intelligence and longevity, which in all likelihood are encoded in complex constellations of multiple genes. If this turns out to be the case, then the trajectory of human genetic enhancement may be one in which the first thing to happen is that the lot of the genetically worst-off is radically improved, through the elimination of diseases such as Tay Sachs, Lesch-Nyhan, Down Syndrome, and early-onset Alzheimer's disease. This would have a major leveling effect on inequalities, not primarily in the monetary sense, but with respect to the even more fundamental parameters of basic opportunities and quality of life.

> *"Unrestrained, HGE [human genetic engineering] is perfectly capable of producing [a] dystopia. . . . We need an international ban on HGE and cloning."*

Human Genetic Engineering Is Risky and Should Be Stopped

David King

In the following viewpoint, David King contends that human genetic engineering is a threat to future generations. King states that genetic engineering is a risky endeavor with no assurance of safety. Although King is sympathetic to those who would use genetic engineering to alleviate sickness, he maintains that tinkering with genes would eventually lead to purely cosmetic enhancements. Once this occurs, King asserts, the future would be dictated by eugenics principles and market forces, leading to a loss of humanity and widening the divide between the haves and the have-nots. David King is a former biologist and the director of Human Genetics Alert, a United Kingdom watchdog organization opposed to human genetic engineering.

David King, "The Threat of Human Genetic Engineering," Human Genetics Alert. www.hgalert.org/topics/hge/threat.htm. Reproduced by permission of the author.

As you read, consider the following questions:

1. What does King see as the first step toward justifying a future dominated by human genetic engineering?

2. In the author's view, what form of genetic engineering illustrates that the practice will never achieve zero risk?

3. How does King use current experiments with human growth hormone to support his claim that human genetic engineering will inevitably lead to cosmetic enhancements?

The main debate around human genetics currently centres on the ethics of genetic testing, and possibilities for genetic discrimination and selective eugenics [the science of controlled or selective improvement of the hereditary qualities of a race or group of people]. But while ethicists and the media constantly re-hash these issues, a small group of scientists and publicists are working towards an even more frightening prospect: the intentional genetic engineering of human beings. Just as [English embryologist] Ian Wilmut presented us with the first clone of an adult mammal, Dolly [a sheep], as a fait accompli, so these scientists aim to set in place the tools of a new techno-eugenics, before the public has ever had a chance to decide whether this is the direction we want to go in. The publicists, meanwhile are trying to convince us that these developments are inevitable. The Campaign Against Human Genetic Engineering has been set up in response to this threat.

A Pressing Threat

Currently, genetic engineering is only applied to non-reproductive cells (this is known as 'gene therapy') in order to treat diseases in a single patient, rather than in all their descendants. Gene therapy is still very unsuccessful, and we are often told that the prospect of reproductive genetic engineering is remote. In fact, the basic technologies for human genetic engineering (HGE) have been available for some time and at present are being refined and improved in a number of ways. We should not make the same mistake that was made with cloning, and assume that the issue is one for the far future.

In the first instance, the likely justifications of HGE will be medical. One major step towards reproductive genetic engineering is the proposal by US gene therapy pioneer, French Anderson, to begin doing gene therapy on foetuses, to treat certain genetic diseases. Although not directly targeted at reproductive cells, Anderson's proposed technique poses a relatively high risk that genes will be 'inadvertently' altered in the reproductive cells of the foetus, as well as in the blood cells which he wants to fix. Thus, if he is allowed to go ahead, the descendants of the foetus will be genetically engineered in every cell of their body. Another scientist, James Grifo of New York University, is transferring cell nuclei from the eggs of older to younger women, using similar techniques to those used in cloning. He aims to overcome certain fertility problems, but the result would be babies with three genetic parents, arguably a form of HGE. In addition to the two normal parents, these babies will have mitochondria (gene-containing subcellular bodies which control energy production in cells) from the younger woman.

The Coming of Enhancement

Anderson is a declared advocate of HGE for medical purposes, and was a speaker at a symposium . . . at UCLA, at which advocates of HGE set out their stall. At the symposium, which was attended by nearly 1,000 people, James Watson, of DNA discovery fame, advocated the use of HGE not merely for medical purposes, but for 'enhancement': 'And the other thing, because no one really has the guts to say it, I mean, if we could make better human beings by knowing how to add genes, why shouldn't we do it?'

In his recent book, *Re-Making Eden* (1998), Princeton biologist Lee Silver celebrates the coming future of human 'enhancement', in which the health, appearance, personality, cognitive ability, sensory capacity, and life-span of our children all become artifacts of genetic engineering, literally selected from a catalog. Silver acknowledges that the costs of these technologies will limit their full use to only a small 'elite', so that over time society will segregate into the "GenRich" and the "Naturals":

> "The GenRich—who account for 10 percent of the American population—all carry synthetic genes ... that were created in the laboratory.... All aspects of the economy, the media, the entertainment industry, and the knowledge industry are controlled by members of the GenRich class.... Naturals work as low-paid service providers or as labourers, and their children go to public schools.... If the accumulation of genetic knowledge and advances in genetic enhancement technology continue ... the GenRich class and the Natural class will become ... entirely separate species with no ability to crossbreed, and with as much romantic interest in each other as a current human would have for a chimpanzee."

Silver, another speaker at the UCLA symposium, believes that these trends should not and cannot be stopped, because to do so would infringe on liberty.

The Safety Charade

Most scientists say that what is preventing them from embarking on HGE is the risk that the process will itself generate new mutations, which will be passed on to future generations. Official scientific and ethical bodies tend to rely on this as the basis for forbidding attempts at HGE, rather than any principled opposition to the idea.

In my view, we should not allow ourselves to be lulled into a false sense of security by this argument. Experience

Our Specialness Will Vanish

Now it's crunch time. Faced with a challenge larger than any we've ever faced—the possible quick erosion of human meaning—we need to rally our innate ability to say no. We will be sorely tempted to engineer our kids, but it's a temptation that we need to resist us individuals and to help each other resist as a society.

The choices we face, in fact, will settle this question of specialness once and for all. If we cannot summon our ability to use self-restraint, or if it proves too weak, we will leave our specialness behind forever. Because once we start down the path of turning ourselves into machines, of writing ineradicable programs for our proteins, then there will be no way, and no reason, to turn back. We'll do what our programming indicates, never knowing how much choice we really have. We'll be like obsessive compulsives. For them, some accident of wiring or chemistry has overridden their ability to choose. They feel as if they have no choice. But tough as their condition is, it can yield to the liberating effects of reflection therapy, medicine.

It won't be faulty wiring, though, that robs the engineered of their agency—it will be intentional programming. We'll do what we're supposed to do—we'll be brainy or brawny or pious. We may not feel sad—we won't necessarily want to be liberated from the way we are programmed—but we'll live in a world where our specialness really has vanished.

Bill McKibben, Christian Century, *May 17, 2003.*

with genetically engineered crops, for example, shows that we are unlikely ever to arrive at a situation when we can be sure that the risks are zero. Instead, when scientists are ready to proceed, we will be told that the risks are 'acceptable', compared to the benefits. Meanwhile, there will be people telling us loudly that since they are taking the risks with their children, we have no right to interfere.

An Unnecessary Medical Solution

One of the flaws in the argument of those who support the possibility of HGE for medical purposes is that there seem to be very few good examples where it is the only solution to the medical problem of genetic disease. The main advantage of HGE is said to be the elimination of disease genes from a family. Yet in nearly all cases, existing technologies of prenatal and preimplantation genetic testing of embryos allow the avoidance of actual disease. There are only a few very rare cases where HGE is the only option.

Furthermore, there is always another solution for those couples who are certain to produce a genetically disabled child and cannot, or do not want to deal with this possibility. They can choose not to have children, to adopt a child, or to use donor eggs or sperm. Parenthood is not the only way to create fulfilment through close, intimate and long lasting relationships with children. The question we have to ask is whether we should develop the technology for HGE, in order to satisfy a very small number of people.

The Inevitability of Cosmetic Enhancement

Although the arguments for the first uses of HGE will be medical, in fact the main market for the technology will be 'enhancement'. Once it was available, how would it be possible to ensure that HGE was used for purely medical purposes? The same problem applies to prenatal genetic screening and to somatic gene therapy, and not only are there no accepted criteria for deciding what constitutes a medical condition, but in a free market society there seems to be no convincing mechanism for arriving at such decision. The best answer that conventional medical ethics seems to have is to 'leave it up to the parents', i.e. to market forces.

Existing trends leave little doubt about what to expect. Sophisticated medical technology and medical personnel are already employed in increasingly fashionable cosmetic surgery. Another example is the use of genetically engineered human growth hormone (HGH), developed to remedy the medical condition of growth hormone deficiency. Because of aggressive marketing by its manufacturers, HGH is routinely prescribed in the USA to normal short children with no hormone deficiency. If these pressures already exist, how much stronger will they be for a technology with as great a power to manipulate human life as HGE?

A New Eugenics Movement

Germ line manipulation opens up, for the first time in human history, the possibility of consciously designing human beings, in a myriad of different ways. I am not generally happy about using the concept of playing God, but it is difficult to avoid in this case. The advocates of genetic engineering point out that humans constantly 'play God', in a sense, by interfering with nature. Yet the environmental crisis has forced us to realise that many of the ways we already do this are not wise, destroy the environment and cannot be sustained. Furthermore, HGE is not just a continuation of existing trends. Once we begin to consciously design ourselves, we will have entered a completely new era of human history, in which human subjects, rather than being accepted as they are will become just another kind of object, shaped according to parental whims and market forces.

In essence, the vision of the advocates of HGE is a sanitised version of the old eugenics doctrines, updated for the [present]. Instead of 'elimination of the unfit', HGE is presented as a tool to end, once and for all, the suffering associated with genetic diseases. And in place of 'improving the race', the [present] emphasis is on freedom of choice, where 'reproductive rights' become consumer rights to choose the characteristics of your child. No doubt the resulting eugenic society would be a little less brutal than those of earlier [times]. On the other hand the capabilities of geneticists are much greater now than they were then. Unrestrained, HGE is perfectly capable of producing Lee Silver's dystopia.

In most cases, the public's function with respect to science is to consume its products, or to pay to clean up the mess. But with HGE, there is still time to prevent it, before it becomes reality. We need an international ban on HGE and cloning. There is a good chance this can be achieved, since both are already illegal in many countries. Of course it may be impossible to prevent a scientist, somewhere, from attempting to clone or genetically engineer humans. But there is a great difference between a society which would jail such a scientist and one which would permit HGE to become widespread and respectable. If we fail to act now, we will only have ourselves to blame.

| "Let us act rationally, and legalise human cloning now."

Human Cloning Should Be Legalized

Hugh McLachlan

In the following viewpoint, Hugh McLachlan claims that fears about human cloning do not justify a ban on the practice. Instead, McLachlan maintains that cloning should be legalized to provide opportunities for couples who have no other way to conceive children. He stipulates that uses beyond this application can easily be controlled or outlawed if enough citizens deem them unethical. But McLachlan reiterates that objections to cloning based on horrific predictions of what might happen should not keep cloning illegal. Hugh McLachlan is a professor of bioethics at Glasgow Caledonian University in Scotland and the co-author of From the Womb to the Tomb: Issues in Medical Ethics.

As you read, consider the following questions:

1. How does McLachlan undercut what he sees as the moral objection to cloning?

Hugh McLachlan, "Let's Legalise Cloning," *New Scientist*, vol. 195, no. 2613, July 21, 2007, p. 20. Copyright © 2007 Reed Elsevier Business Publishing, Ltd. Reproduced by permission.

2. What does the author say has had more impact on the human gene pool than cloning ever could?

3. What objection to human cloning, according to McLachlan, is no more reasonable than the claim that "rape is an objection to sex"?

In many countries, including the UK [United Kingdom], human reproductive cloning—creating a baby from the genetic material of a single adult—is a criminal offence. This is not generally seen as controversial: scientific societies, medical groups and governments around the world have condemned the idea of human cloning since the technique was first demonstrated in mammals in 1997.

But why are we so against the idea of cloned human babies? As a bioethicist specialising in reproductive issues, I believe it has more to do with an irrational fear of cloning than any logical reason. All the arguments in favour of a ban describe risks that we accept quite easily and naturally in other areas of reproduction.

Clones Are Not Exact Copies

One argument against human cloning is the idea that it is morally wrong or undesirable to create replicas of people. But although a clone has the same gene set as the adult from which it was cloned, environmental factors will ensure that the resulting individual is not an identical copy, either psychologically or physically. What's more, we accept genetically identical people in the form of twins. If anything, clones would be less alike than twins because they would be different ages and be brought up in different contexts. Objecting to cloning on these grounds makes no sense.

Another key concern is safety. We know from animal cloning studies that the risks to the mother and the baby are likely to be very high, although they may diminish as the technique is perfected. Yet in other areas of reproduction (or life in general) safety alone is not seen as sufficient grounds to make something illegal. The risks should be explained to the prospective mother, and she should then have the right to decide for herself, as with any other medical procedure, whether to accept them.

The potential baby, of course, cannot give consent. There may be an increased risk of miscarriage or being born with a deformity, but for people born as a result of cloning, it is their only chance of life. Cloning is therefore not a risk but an opportunity. If you could only have been born as a clone, with the risks that entails, would you have wanted your life to have been prevented? I would say loudly: no.

We accept this principle for other types of reproduction. Of embryos produced normally, 75 per cent do not make it to birth. Nor do we ban couples who carry disease genes from reproducing, even though their children have a high risk of suffering from a serious disorder—25 per cent for cystic fibrosis, for example. Many such couples choose not to have a child, or to have their embryos screened, but it is their choice.

Cloning Will Remain a Last Resort

Let's address also the idea that legalising cloning would allow fertility clinics to exploit desperate couples. The possibility of exploitation is not seen as a reason to make other forms of assisted reproduction illegal. Instead, we regulate clinics to make sure that patients are told the risks, so they can make their own informed decisions.

Other arguments in favour of banning cloning are more outlandish, such as the idea that it might alter the gene pool, or that despotic leaders might use cloning to create armies of ideal soldiers. These are red herrings. If cloning were legalised it is likely only a tiny percentage of people would take it up. After all, sexual reproduction remains cheaper, safer and more fun: only those with no other option are likely to resort to cloning.

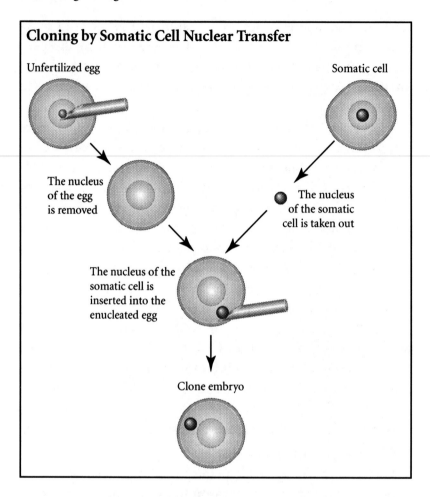

Cloning by Somatic Cell Nuclear Transfer

Unfertilized egg

Somatic cell

The nucleus of the egg is removed

The nucleus of the somatic cell is taken out

The nucleus of the somatic cell is inserted into the enucleated egg

Clone embryo

Even if growing numbers of clones could affect the gene pool, is that a reason for making the practice illegal? It's not as though there is any "natural" or preordained path along which our species is meant to develop. Global travel has presumably had a far greater effect on the gene pool than cloning ever could, and nobody uses that to argue for a ban on it.

Potential for Misuse Not Grounds for Outlawing

As for state-run cloning factories, any organised programme to rear babies for a particular purpose would clearly be abhorrent, whether the children were produced by sexual intercourse, IVF [in vitro fertilization] or cloning. This has no bearing on whether individual couples should be allowed to choose cloning as a method by which to have a child. Similarly, if someone was cloned without their consent, that would be unethical and should be illegal, but it is not a reasonable objection to cloning any more than rape is an objection to sex.

In a free society, actions should be legal unless there is a case for making them illegal. We do not need to justify cloning in order to say that it should be legal (although it would clearly benefit those infertile couples for whom there is no other way to have a child that is genetically related to them). It should be for those who want cloning to remain a crime to justify themselves.

The trouble with the arguments given in favour of a ban is that when we look closely, they turn out to be irrational and inconsistent. They describe risks that we accept—and are right to accept—in other methods of reproduction. Let us act rationally, and legalise human cloning now.

> *"The dismal results of animal cloning have convinced many scientists that it is unthinkable to clone a human."*

Human Cloning Should Be Banned

Wendy Wright

In the following viewpoint, Wendy Wright argues that human reproductive cloning creates a culture in which people are viewed as replaceable and controllable. She believes that the poor results obtained from animal cloning experiments should convince rational people that the technology is unpredictable and dangerous. Wright also dismisses therapeutic cloning by asserting that stem cell research has already proven that noncloned adult stem cells can work wonders with genetic diseases, making cloning unnecessary. Wendy Wright is the president of Concerned Women for America, the nation's largest women's public policy organization. A pro-life spokesperson, Wright is a frequent lobbyist before the United Nations as well as the U.S. Congress on women's rights, cloning, and human rights issues.

As you read, consider the following questions:

1. As Wright describes, what resulted from the experiments on monkey embryos conducted by Dr. Tanja Dominko?

Wendy Wright, "Cloning: Medical Miracle or Human Hubris?" Concerned Women for America, June 17, 2003. www.cwfa.org. Reproduced by permission.

2. What are some of the medical problems that Wright says accompany the birth of cloned cows, sheep, goats, and mice?

3. Why does the author contend that a ban on reproductive cloning alone will not work?

Cloning is the creation of a being that is genetically identical to its "parent." The common method, used with Dolly the sheep, is to extract the nucleus from an egg, inject a cell containing DNA from the donor, and then give the egg a shock of electricity to stimulate cell division.

In "reproductive cloning," the new life is implanted in a surrogate mother and allowed to grow and be born. "Therapeutic cloning" uses the same method, but rather than implanting the clone and allowing it to be born, researchers use the embryo as raw material for experiments or to scavenge for parts, such as skin, muscle, nerve or brain cells. A "therapeutic clone" is no different from a "reproductive clone"—only the researchers' intent on what to do with the clone changes.

The goal of therapeutic cloning is to obtain embryonic stem cells that, in theory, may develop into any kind of cell or body tissue. Scientists hope to use the stem cells to treat diseases. Since the embryo's tissue would be genetically identical to the donor, it could conceivably avoid the problem of tissue rejection. However, in animals, it often takes 100 or more eggs to get one viable clone. (After receiving hormone injections for days for in vitro fertilization, women will typically produce 10 to 15 eggs.) Further, the success of these treatments is speculative. No disease or disability in humans has yet been cured through the use of embryonic stem cells.

High Failure Rate of Cloning

Advanced Cell Technology [ACT], a Massachusetts bio-tech firm, claims it created one human embryo that grew into six cells before dying. Embryonic stem cells are not present at this early stage. Most of the eggs in the research died without dividing once. Despite the headlines that a human clone had been created, objective researchers noted there was more hype than substance behind the announcement, perhaps to gain attention and funding for the bio-tech firm.

Regardless, Dr. Tanja Dominko, an Advanced Cell Technology researcher, said her work on cloning monkey embryos (before she joined ACT) resulted in gross abnormalities in most embryos, which died within five days—too early for stem cells to appear. Though they look healthy, Dr. Dominko said, a high percentage of cloned monkey embryos are really a "gallery of horrors" within.

Most efforts fail, even in species that have at one time or another been cloned. Researchers who have occasional success cloning one species, like cows, are finding failure with others, like dogs. Cloning success is the exception, not the rule.

Dr. [Ian] Wilmut, the British scientist who successfully cloned Dolly the sheep, said, in general, just 1 to 4 percent of efforts *in a species where cloning has worked* result in the birth of a live animal. That, he said, indicates that cloning appears to create serious abnormalities in almost all embryos.

Severe problems, including defects in the heart, lungs and other organs, are suffered by half of all clones of large mammals, like sheep and cows. Most die before they are born. Others that survive die suddenly and mysteriously weeks or months after birth.

Cloning Defies Human Uniqueness

While reproductive cloning of humans is nearly universally condemned, rogue scientists and their benefactors continue to attempt it. Rep. Dave Weldon's (R-Florida) "Human Cloning Prohibition Act of 2001" (H.R. 2505) would ban all human cloning, while permitting the replication of DNA, cells or tissues (but not embryos) for experimental or therapeutic purposes. It passed in the House of Representatives, but Majority

Cloning by Any Other Name . . .

I, along with the president [George W. Bush] and the vast majority of Americans, do not believe that we should create human life just to destroy it—yet that is exactly what is being proposed by those who support cloning in some circumstances. However they might name the procedure—whether they call it nuclear transplantation, therapeutic cloning, therapeutic cellular transfer, DNA regenerative therapy or some other euphemism—it is simply human cloning.

Sam Brownback, National Review, *February 26, 2003.*

Leader Tom Daschle (D-South Dakota) continues to delay a vote in the Senate. [It failed to pass the Senate, and subsequent bills have also stalled in Congress.]

The United Nations condemned reproductive cloning in 1997 when it unanimously adopted the Universal Declaration on the Human Genome and Human Rights. This states, "Practices which are contrary to human dignity, such as reproductive cloning of human beings, shall not be permitted." In 2000, the United Kingdom passed a ban on reproductive cloning, but allowed for therapeutic cloning.

This revulsion for the cloning of humans is a natural response to the utter disregard for human dignity. Cloning inherently treats people as "replacements" or "extras." This defies the uniqueness of each individual, using technology to manipulate and control human beings. It would create a class of humans deprived of a clear identity, parents and family.

Scientists who claim to be helping grieving family or friends by resurrecting a loved one through cloning are committing fraud. Experiments to create cloned humans carry unimagined, horrific physical risks to the clone and to the woman who carries it. Most animal embryo clones are horribly deformed and die. The few that live long enough to be implanted in an animal's uterus die soon afterward. The anomalies that have survived to birth are prone to genetic defects. A cloned lamb born soon after Dolly displayed such severe respiratory problems that within a few weeks she was euthanized. An autopsy revealed that her lungs had not developed properly.

Cloned cows, sheep, goats, and mice often have over-sized internal organs, limbs, and overall body, and the newborns are sickly. The large fetuses cause a risk to the mother during delivery. The dismal results of animal cloning have convinced many scientists that it is unthinkable to clone a human.

Beyond the physical problems, the cloned human has no defined rights. Who is the parent—the donor or the scientist? Who is responsible when things go wrong? Could a cloned human be killed if he or she were found to be defective or unwanted? Would a clone be treated differently than humans with two biological parents? When would a clone have legal or human rights? What if a living or deceased person is cloned without his or her knowledge or consent?

It is wrong to treat a human as something that can be replaced, and it is wrong to treat another human as a mere substitute.

Therapeutic Cloning Is Also Flawed

Therapeutic cloning, or creating clones to harvest their cells, was also roundly condemned until scientists and their fundraisers promoted the idea that the end (helping patients) justifies the means (creating humans to use for experiments or parts).

However, cloned (or even adult) stem cells would not be useful unless the genetic defects were corrected before they were injected back into a patient. "It's one thing to re-create a pancreas, but if you have to regenerate from diseased tissue, the gene is still defective," says Inder M. Verma of the Salk Institute for Biological Studies in San Diego, California. "You have to correct the defect; otherwise cloning will get you what you started out with."

There Is Hope for Patients

Since the excuse for allowing scientists to pursue therapeutic cloning is to obtain valuable stem cells, if there are other—or better—sources for stem cells, then the dangers and indignities of cloning cannot be justified. And, there are much better sources.

Stem cells from adults and umbilical cord blood are already being used to treat numerous kinds of cancer and diseases, to regenerate muscle tissue, and to form cartilage and bone tissue. Adult stem cells bypass the problem of donor rejection, as the patient is the donor, and are a quicker source for stem cells than the laborious, unnecessary step of creating an embryo. There is no need to go through the immoral and dangerous process of cloning when stem cells can be safely obtained directly from the patient. . . .

Partial Ban Will Not Work

Sen. Tom Daschle (D-South Dakota) and other politicians say they support a ban on reproductive cloning, but not a ban on therapeutic. Both the United Nations' resolution and England's ban allow for therapeutic cloning. But can a partial ban work?

The only way to uphold such a ban would be to forcefully abort a woman carrying a human clone. Barring that, how would politicians deal with a clone who escapes detection and is born? Since the clone had no right to be born, would this new person have any legal or human rights, or even be recognized as a human being?

Those working on the front lines recognize that the demarcation between reproductive and therapeutic cloning is easy to cross. Advanced Cell Technology's president Michael West, while arguing for therapeutic cloning, has written that reproductive cloning is "unwarranted at this time" and should be restricted—that is, "until the safety and ethical issues surrounding it are resolved."

Severino Antinori, a scientist who claims he will create a cloned human being soon, stated that reproductive cloning is therapeutic cloning. He argues that infertility is a disease, and the cure, or therapy, is cloning.

Cloning Is High-Tech Slavery

Cloning causes people to view human beings as commodities, something to be mass-produced. Cloning supporters attempt to imitate God, but their intentions are warped from His because they desire to produce beings that are distinctly *not* unique. If clones were distinct, individual, one-of-a-kind— traits of all humans, including identical twins—the goal of cloning supporters would be thwarted. Noble excuses cannot disguise the reprehensible mindset that views human beings as replaceable.

Slavery treats a class of people as sub-human. Depraved philosophies like that of the Nazi experimenters view people only in the context of how their body parts can be exploited. Cloning is the modern-day version of history's corrupt endeavors. The act of cloning views human life as something to be manipulated, used, and disposed of. It endangers the life and health of the offspring, most of which will die in the process, while the few survivors will have deformities and suffer indignities. If we allow technology and rogue scientists to determine the worth, relationships and use of people, civilization as we know it will suffer.

> "We need to allow . . . research using only those embryonic stem cells . . . that are left over after in vitro fertilization and would otherwise be discarded."

Human Embryos Destined for Discard Should Be Used for Research

Bill Frist

In the following viewpoint, physician and former U.S. senator from Tennessee Bill Frist tells the Senate why he supports embryonic stem cell research. According to Frist, embryonic stem cells offer potential cures to debilitating genetic diseases. These miraculous cures, in Frist's view, will not likely come from adult stem cells because these cells have less resilient capacities and limited medical uses. Although Frist is pro-life, he argues that losing nascent human life in discarded embryonic stem cells is preferable when compared to the possibilities of treating or eradicating diseases in the larger population. For these reasons Frist advocates overturning current policies of the George W. Bush administration that limit funding for embryonic stem cell research. Bill Frist retired from his Senate post in 2007 and returned to practicing medicine.

Bill Frist, comments on stem cell research to the U.S. Senate, July 29, 2005.

As you read, consider the following questions:

1. How does Frist propose to regulate the use of only discarded embryos in stem cell research?

2. According to the author, what does it mean when embryonic stem cells are referred to as pluripotent?

3. In what way might adult stem cells be reprogrammed to obviate the need for embryonic research, in Frist's opinion?

I came to [the U.S. Senate] floor [in 2001] and laid out a comprehensive proposal to promote stem cell research within a thorough framework of ethics. I proposed 10 specific interdependent principles. They dealt with all types of stem cell research, including adult and embryonic stem cells.

As we know, adult stem cell research is not controversial on ethical grounds—while embryonic stem cell research is. Right now, to derive embryonic stem cells, an embryo—which many, including myself, consider nascent human life—must be destroyed. But I also strongly believe—as do countless other scientists, clinicians, and doctors—that embryonic stem cells uniquely hold specific promise for some therapies and potential cures that adult stem cells cannot provide.

I'll come back to that later. Right now, though, let me say this: I believe today—as I believed and stated in 2001, prior to the establishment of current policy [which prohibits government funding of most embryonic stem cell research]—that the federal government should fund embryonic stem cell research. And as I said [then], we should federally fund research only on embryonic stem cells derived from blastocysts leftover from fertility therapy, which will not be implanted or adopted but instead are otherwise destined by the parents with absolute certainty to be discarded and destroyed.

Use Only Discarded Embryos

Let me read to you my 5th principle as I presented it on this floor [in 2001]:

No. 5. Provide funding for embryonic stem cell research only from blastocysts that would otherwise be discarded. We need to allow Federal funding for research using only those embryonic stem cells derived from blastocysts that are left over after in vitro fertilization and would otherwise be discarded (Cong. Rec. 18 July 2001: S7847).

I made it clear at the time, and do so again today, that such funding should only be provided within a system of comprehensive ethical oversight. Federally funded embryonic research should be allowed only with transparent and fully informed consent of the parents. And that consent should be granted under a careful and thorough federal regulatory system, which considers both science and ethics. Such a comprehensive ethical system, I believe, is absolutely essential. Only with strict safeguards, public accountability, and complete transparency will we ensure that this new, evolving research unfolds within accepted ethical bounds. . . .

In all forms of stem cell research, I see today, just as I saw in 2001, great promise to heal. Whether it's diabetes, Parkinson's disease, heart disease, Lou Gehrig's disease, or spinal cord injuries, stem cells offer hope for treatment that other lines of research cannot offer.

Embryonic stem cells have specific properties that make them uniquely powerful and deserving of special attention in the realm of medical science. These special properties explain why scientists and physicians feel so strongly about support of embryonic as well as adult stem cell research.

Unlike other stem cells, embryonic stem cells are "pluripotent." That means they have the capacity to become any type of tissue in the human body. Moreover, they are capable of renewing themselves and replicating themselves over and over again—indefinitely.

Adult stem cells meet certain medical needs. But embryonic stem cells—because of these unique characteristics—meet other medical needs that simply cannot be met today by

Diverse Stem Cell Lines Needed

Imagine trying to establish a national blood bank and being restricted to using only Type B+ blood. That is the exact problem our nation's population faces under the current federal embryonic stem cell research policy.

One goal of embryonic stem cell research is to replace diseased cells with functioning ones created from stem cell lines—for example, insulin secreting cells for diabetes or dopamine-producing nerve cells for Parkinson's disease. Since the recipients of these potentially life-saving therapies will come from diverse genetic backgrounds, it is essential that the stem cell lines also possess genetic diversity.

Yet, with only 22 embryonic stem cell lines available for federally funded research, the possibilities of studying, discovering and eventually applying therapies to a genetically-diverse population is severely limited. The current number of lines cannot possibly represent the required genetic diversity to be able to develop potential therapies for all Americans.

Juvenile Diabetes Research Foundation International,
September 21, 2004.

adult stem cells. They especially offer hope for treating a range of diseases that require tissue to regenerate or restore function.

The Current Limited Policy

On August 9, 2001, shortly after I outlined my principles (Cong. Rec. 18 July 2001: S7846–S7851), President [George W.] Bush announced his policy on embryonic stem cell research. His policy was fully consistent with my . . . principles, so I strongly supported it. It federally funded embryonic stem cell research for the first time. It did so within an ethical framework. And it showed respect for human life.

But this policy restricted embryonic stem cell funding only to those cell lines that had been derived from embryos before the date of his announcement. In my policy I, too, proposed restricting the number of cell lines, but I did not propose a specific cutoff date. Over time, with a limited number of cell lines, would we be able to realize the full promise of embryonic stem cell research?

When the President announced his policy, it was widely believed that 78 embryonic stem cell lines would be available for federal funding. That has proven not to be the case. Today only 22 lines are eligible. Moreover, those lines unexpectedly after several generations are starting to become less stable and less replicative than initially thought (they are acquiring and losing chromosomes, losing the normal karyotype, and potentially losing growth control). They also were grown on mouse feeder cells, which we have learned since, will likely limit their future potential for clinical therapy in humans (e.g., potential of viral contamination).

While human embryonic stem cell research is still at a very early stage, the limitations put in place in 2001 will, over time, slow our ability to bring potential new treatments for certain diseases. Therefore, I believe the President's policy should be modified. We should expand federal funding (and thus NIH [National Institutes of Health] oversight) and current guidelines governing stem cell research, carefully and thoughtfully staying within ethical bounds. . . .

Bridging Faith and Science

I am pro-life. I believe human life begins at conception. It is at this moment that the organism is complete—yes, immature—but complete. An embryo is nascent human life. It's genetically distinct. And it's biologically human. It's living. This position is consistent with my faith. But, to me, it isn't just a matter of faith. It's a fact of science.

Our development is a continuous process—gradual and chronological. We were all once embryos. The embryo is human life at its earliest stage of development. And accordingly, the human embryo has moral significance and moral worth. It deserves to be treated with the utmost dignity and respect.

I also believe that embryonic stem cell research should be encouraged and supported. But, just as I said in 2001, it should advance in a manner that affords all human life dignity and respect—the same dignity and respect we bring to the table as we work with children and adults to advance the frontiers of medicine and health.

Promoting Alternatives

Congress must have the ability to fully exercise its oversight authority on an ongoing basis. And policymakers, I believe, have a responsibility to re-examine stem cell research policy in the future and, if necessary, make adjustments.

This is essential, in no small part, because of promising research not even imagined [in 2001]. Exciting techniques are now emerging that may make it unnecessary to destroy embryos (even those that will be discarded anyway) to obtain cells with the same unique "pluripotential" properties as embryonic stem cells.

For example, an adult stem cell could be "reprogrammed" back to an earlier embryonic stage. This, in particular, may prove to be the best way, both scientifically and ethically, to overcome rejection and other barriers to effective stem cell therapies. To me—and I would hope to every member of this body [the Senate]—that's research worth supporting. Shouldn't we want to discover therapies and cures—given a choice—through the most ethical and moral means?

So let me make it crystal clear: I strongly support newer, alternative means of deriving, creating, and isolating pluripotent stem cells—whether they're true embryonic stem cells or stem cells that have all of the unique properties of embryonic stem cells.

With more federal support and emphasis, these newer methods, though still preliminary today, may offer huge scientific and clinical pay-offs. And just as important, they may bridge moral and ethical differences among people who now hold very different views on stem cell research because they totally avoid destruction of any human embryos.

| "Some people argue that finding new cures for disease requires the destruction of human embryos. . . . I disagree."

Human Embryos Destined for Discard Should Not Be Used for Research

George W. Bush

In the following viewpoint, George W. Bush, the 43rd president of the United States, defends his reasons for not signing legislation that would allow government funding of embryonic stem cell research in which embryos are destroyed. Bush maintains that human life is valuable and that embryos discarded from in vitro fertilization are nascent human life. Thus, he would not see these embryos harvested for stem cells and then terminated. Furthermore, Bush claims that America's moral conscience would not support such disregard for human life. Instead, Bush proposes that America should research and fund alternatives to embryonic experiments.

As you read, consider the following questions:

1. According to Bush, how many embryonic stem cell lines are already sanctioned for research?

George W. Bush, President Discusses Stem Cell Research Policy, July 19, 2006. www .whitehouse.gov.

2. As the author explains, why did the Alternative Pluripotent Stem Cell Therapies Enhancement Act fail to pass Congress?

3. According to Bush, what bill—if not vetoed—would have compelled American taxpayers to fund the deliberate destruction of human embryos?

Congress has just [in 2006] passed and sent to my desk two bills concerning the use of stem cells in biomedical research. These bills illustrate both the promise and perils we face in the age of biotechnology. In this new era, our challenge is to harness the power of science to ease human suffering without sanctioning the practices that violate the dignity of human life.

In 2001, I spoke to the American people and set forth a new policy on stem cell research that struck a balance between the needs of science and the demands of conscience. When I took office, there was no federal funding for human embryonic stem cell research. Under the policy I announced [in 2001], my administration became the first to make federal funds available for this research, yet only on embryonic stem cell lines derived from embryos that had already been destroyed.

My administration has made available more than $90 million for research on these lines. This policy has allowed important research to go forward without using taxpayer funds to encourage the further deliberate destruction of human embryos.

One of the bills Congress has passed [i.e., the Fetus Farming Prohibition Act] builds on the progress we have made [since then]. So I signed it into law. Congress has also passed a second bill [i.e., the Stem Cell Research Enhancement Act] that attempts to overturn the balanced policy I set. This bill would support the taking of innocent human life in the hope of finding medical benefits for others. It crosses a moral boundary that our decent society needs to respect, so I vetoed it.

Embryos Are Not Spare Parts

Like all Americans, I believe our nation must vigorously pursue the tremendous possibility that science offers to cure disease and improve the lives of millions. We have opportunities to discover cures and treatments that were unthinkable generations ago. Some scientists believe that one source of these cures might be embryonic stem cell research. Embryonic stem cells have the ability to grow into specialized adult tissues, and this may give them the potential to replace damaged or defective cells or body parts and treat a variety of diseases.

Yet we must also remember that embryonic stem cells come from human embryos that are destroyed for their cells. Each of these human embryos is a unique human life with inherent dignity and matchless value. We see that value in the children who are with us [in the East Room of the White House] today. Each of these children began his or her life as a frozen embryo that was created for in vitro fertilization, but remained unused after the fertility treatments were complete. Each of these children was adopted while still an embryo, and has been blessed with the chance to grow up in a loving family.

These boys and girls are not spare parts. They remind us of what is lost when embryos are destroyed in the name of research. They remind us that we all begin our lives as a small collection of cells. And they remind us that in our zeal for new treatments and cures, America must never abandon our fundamental morals.

Matching Science with Ethics

Some people argue that finding new cures for disease requires the destruction of human embryos like the ones that these families adopted. I disagree. I believe that with the right tech-

The Answer Is: No

So should our tax dollars be spent on embryonic stem cell research? The answer is: No. The scientific data on embryonic stem cell research simply do not support the continued investment in research. Many researchers have failed. Even private investors are not backing this, and that is a strong indication of the lack of success. Even if it was successful, it is clear that embryonic stem cell research is morally bankrupt and endangers women, while adult stem cell research doesn't present any of these problems.

Kelly Hollowell,
Heritage Foundation Lecture #888,
June 24, 2005.

niques and the right policies, we can achieve scientific progress while living up to our ethical responsibilities. That's what I sought in 2001, when I set forth my administration's policy allowing federal funding for research on embryonic stem cell lines where the life and death decision had already been made.

This balanced approach has worked. Under this policy, 21 human embryonic stem cell lines are currently in use in research that is eligible for federal funding. Each of these lines can be replicated many times. And as a result, the National Institutes of Health have helped make more than 700 shipments to researchers since 2001. There is no ban on embryonic stem cell research. To the contrary, even critics of my policy concede that these federally funded lines are being used in research every day by scientists around the world. My policy has allowed us to explore the potential of embryonic stem cells, and it has allowed America to continue to lead the world in this area.

Since I announced my policy in 2001, advances in scientific research have also shown the great potential of stem calls that are derived without harming human embryos. My administration has expanded the funding of research into stem cells that can be drawn from children, adults, and the blood in umbilical cords, with no harm to the donor. And these stem cells are already being used in medical treatments.

With us today [in the East Room] are patients who have benefited from treatments with adult and umbilical-cord-blood stem cells. And I want to thank you all for coming.

They are living proof that effective medical science can also be ethical. Researchers are now also investigating new techniques that could allow doctors and scientists to produce stem cells just as versatile as those derived from human embryos. One technique scientists are exploring would involve reprogramming an adult cell. For example, a skin cell to function like an embryonic stem cell. Science offers the hope that we may one day enjoy the potential benefits of embryonic stem cells without destroying human life.

Holding Back Important Legislation

We must continue to explore these hopeful alternatives and advance the cause of scientific research while staying true to the ideals of a decent and humane society. The bill I sign today upholds these humane ideals and draws an important ethical line to guide our research. The Fetus Farming Prohibition Act was sponsored by Senators [Rick] Santorum and [Sam] Brownback—both who are here. And by Congressman Dave Weldon, along with Nathan Deal. Thank you, Congressmen. This good law prohibits one of the most egregious abuses in biomedical research, the trafficking in human fetuses that are created with the sole intent of aborting them to harvest their parts. Human beings are not a raw material to be exploited, or a commodity to be bought or sold, and this bill will help ensure that we respect the fundamental ethical line.

I'm disappointed that Congress failed to pass another bill [i.e., the Alternative Pluripotent Stem Cell Therapies Enhancement Act] that would have promoted good research. This bill was sponsored by Senator Santorum and Senator Arlen Specter and Congressman Roscoe Bartlett.... It would have authorized additional federal funding for promising new research that could produce cells with the abilities of embryonic cells, but without the destruction of human embryos. This is an important piece of legislation. This bill was unanimously approved by the Senate; it received 273 votes in the House of Representatives, but was blocked by a minority in the House using procedural maneuvers. I'm disappointed that the House failed to authorize funding for this vital and ethical research.

It makes no sense to say that you're in favor of finding cures for terrible diseases as quickly as possible, and then block a bill that would authorize funding for promising and ethical stem cell research. At a moment when ethical alternatives are becoming available, we cannot lose the opportunity to conduct research that would give hope to those suffering from terrible diseases, and help move our nation beyond the current controversies over embryonic stem cell research.

We must pursue this research. And so I direct the Secretary of Health and Human Services, Secretary [Mike] Leavitt, and the Director of the National Institutes of Health to use all the tools at their disposal to aid the search for stem cell techniques that advance promising medical science in an ethical and morally responsible way. Unfortunately, Congress has sent me a bill that fails to meet this ethical test. This legislation would overturn the balanced policy on embryonic stem cell research that my administration has followed [since 2001]. This bill would also undermine the principle that Congress, itself, has followed for more than a decade, when it has prohibited federal funding for research that destroys human embryos.

If this bill would have become law, American taxpayers would, for the first time in our history, be compelled to fund the deliberate destruction of human embryos. And I'm not going to allow it.

Resisting Temptation

I made it clear to the Congress that I will not allow our nation to cross this moral line. I felt like crossing this line would be a mistake, and once crossed, we would find it almost impossible to turn back. Crossing the line would needlessly encourage a conflict between science and ethics that can only do damage to both, and to our nation as a whole. If we're to find the right ways to advance ethical medical research, we must also be willing, when necessary, to reject the wrong ways. So today, I'm keeping the promise I made to the American people by returning this bill to Congress with my veto.

As science brings us ever closer to unlocking the secrets of human biology, it also offers temptations to manipulate human life and violate human dignity. Our conscience and history as a nation demand that we resist this temptation. America was founded on the principle that we are all created equal, and endowed by our Creator with the right to life. We can advance the cause of science while upholding this founding promise. We can harness the promise of technology without becoming slaves to technology. And we can ensure that science serves the cause of humanity instead of the other way around.

America pursues medical advances in the name of life, and we will achieve the great breakthroughs we all seek with reverence for the gift of life. I believe America's scientists have the ingenuity and skill to meet this challenge. And I look forward to working with Congress and the scientific community to achieve these great and noble goals in the years ahead.

Periodical Bibliography

The following articles have been selected to supplement the diverse views presented in this chapter.

American Spectator	"No, the Stem Cell Debate Is Not Over," April 2008.
Donald Bruce	"Over-Egging the Clones," *New Scientist*, January 20, 2007.
David Epstein	"The Future," *Sports Illustrated*, March 17, 2008.
James Harkin	"A Plastic People Future," *New Statesman*, November 20, 2006.
Horace Freeland Judson	"The Glimmering Promise of Gene Therapy," *Technology Review*, November 2006.
Bruno Maddox	"Blinded by Science," *Discover*, November 2006.
Richard Monastersky	"Stem-Cell Advances Could Speed Research," *Chronicle of Higher Education*, November 30, 2007.
Neil Munro	"Cloning Critics Split," *National Journal*, February 2, 2008.
National Review	"Stem-Cell Success," December 17, 2007.
New Scientist	"The Point of No Return," November 18, 2006.
David S. Oderberg	"Human Embryonic Stem Cell Research: What's Wrong with It?" *Human Life Review*, Fall 2005.
Alice Park	"Man Makes Life," *Time*, February 4, 2008.
Virginia Postrel	"Criminalizing Science," *Forbes*, October 17, 2005.
Christine Soares	"Ancient Gene, New Tricks," *Scientific American*, July 2008.

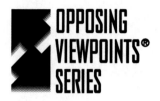

CHAPTER 2

Is Genetic Engineering Ethical?

Chapter Preface

The issue of embryonic stem cell research has created considerable ethical controversy because some people regard it as experimenting on human life. Because of this, scientists have been seeking creative alternatives to obtain the embryonic stem cells that are vital to their research. One innovative process is to create a parthenote—an egg that is triggered into becoming an embryo without fertilization. In this process, an unfertilized egg can be coaxed into cellular division and organization through the use of a chemical trigger. This chemical trigger tricks the egg into thinking it has been fertilized.

Parthenotes generate stem cells but cannot develop beyond the early embryonic stage because of their genetic programming. Critics of this type of experimentation claim, however, that it is unclear whether the immature parthenote can be considered a form of human life. As William P. Cheshire, an assistant professor of neurology at the Mayo Clinic, explains, "Though it is a profoundly defective and abbreviated life, yet it may still be a human life with special dignity science cannot measure."

Cheshire further contends that because the parthenote is a stunted embryo, its stem cells may not be as mature as its fertilized counterparts. In his view, this may render them useless in genetic therapies. He concedes that genetic engineering may be able to correct this shortcoming, but he maintains that this might make them more like fertilized embryos and thus "betray a false moral distinction as improved generations of parthenotes [come] to resemble more and more the traditional human embryo in their capacity for fullness of life." For such reasons, Cheshire opposes experimentation on parthenotes until it can be conclusively proven that these embryos are not nascent human life.

In the following chapter, various authors contend with the ethical issues that surround the manipulation of genetic material. Of those who discuss tampering with the human genome, some maintain that other options exist that make embryonic research unnecessary. Others, however, believe that to ignore such avenues of research is to condemn many people to live under the burden of genetic diseases that otherwise might be cured through embryonic research.

> *"Defenders of enhancement argue that there is no difference, in principle, between improving children through education and improving them through bioengineering. Critics of enhancement insist there is all the difference in the world."*

Genetic Engineering Is Unethical

Michael J. Sandel

In the following viewpoint, Michael J. Sandel argues that genetic enhancement—when used to modify children—disrupts the relationship between parents and child. Sandel claims that parents learn lessons of humility and sympathy from raising children that act unpredictably or do not always meet parental expectations. Genetic enhancement, in his view, would eliminate that human experience because children would be molded into exactly what parents deem acceptable. Michael J. Sandel teaches

Michael J. Sandel, "Designer Children, Designing Parents," in *The Case Against Perfection: Ethics in the Age of Genetic Engineering*. Cambridge, MA: The Belknap Press of Harvard University Press, 2007. Copyright © 2007 by the President and Fellows of Harvard College. All rights reserved. Reproduced by permission of Harvard University Press.

political philosophy at Harvard University. He is the author of The Case against Perfection: Ethics in the Age of Genetic Engineering, *from which the following viewpoint is taken.*

As you read, consider the following questions:

1. What is meant by the phrase "openness to the unbidden," which Sandel quotes in his essay?
2. What value does good health have other than the instrumental value assigned to it by those in favor of genetic modification of children?
3. What are the two types of love that Sandel says parents have for their children? How does he use them to further his argument?

The ethic of giftedness, under siege in sports, persists in the practice of parenting. But here, too, bioengineering and genetic enhancement threaten to dislodge it. To appreciate children as gifts is to accept them as they come, not as objects of our design, or products of our will, or instruments of our ambition. Parental love is not contingent on the talents and attributes the child happens to have. We choose our friends and spouses at least partly on the basis of qualities we find attractive. But we do not choose our children. Their qualities are unpredictable, and even the most conscientious parents cannot be held wholly responsible for the kind of child they have. That is why parenthood, more than other human relationships, teaches what the theologian William F. May calls an "openness to the unbidden."

Molding and Beholding

May's resonant phrase describes a quality of character and heart that restrains the impulse to mastery and control and prompts a sense of life as gift. It helps us see that the deepest moral objection to enhancement lies less in the perfection it seeks than in the human disposition it expresses and promotes. The problem is not that the parents usurp the autonomy of the child they design. (It is not as if the child could otherwise choose her genetic traits for herself.) The problem lies in the hubris of the designing parents, in their drive to master the mystery of birth. Even if this disposition does not make parents tyrants to their children, it disfigures the relation between parent and child, and deprives the parent of the humility and enlarged human sympathies that an openness to the unbidden can cultivate.

To appreciate children as gifts or blessings is not to be passive in the face of illness or disease. Healing a sick or injured child does not override her natural capacities but permits them to flourish. Although medical treatment intervenes in nature, it does so for the sake of health, and so does not represent a boundless bid for mastery and dominion. Even strenuous attempts to treat or cure disease do not constitute a Promethean assault on the given. The reason is that medicine is governed, or at least guided, by the norm of restoring and preserving the natural human functions that constitute health.

Medicine, like sports, is a practice with a purpose, a telos, that orients and constraints it. Of course what counts as good health or normal human functioning is open to argument; it is not only a biological question. People disagree, for example, about whether deafness is a disability to be cured or a form of community and identity to be cherished. But even the disagreement proceeds from the assumption that the point of medicine is to promote health and cure disease.

Some people argue that a parent's obiligation to heal a sick child implies an obligation to enhance a healthy one, to maximize his or her potential for success in life. But this is true only if one accepts the utilitarian idea that health is not a distinctive human good, but simply a means of maximizing happiness or well-being. Bioethicist Julian Savulescu argues, for example, that "health is not intrinsically valuable," only "instrumentally valuable," a "resource" that allows us to do what we want. This way of thinking about health rejects the distinction between healing and enhancing. According to Savulescu, parents not only have a duty to promote their children's health; they are also "morally obliged to genetically modify their children." Parents should use technology to manipulate their children's "memory, temperament, patience, empathy, sense of humor, optimism," and other characteristics in order to give them "the best opportunity of the best life."

But it is a mistake to think of health in wholly instrumental terms, as a way of maximizing something else. Good health, like good character, is a constitutive element of human flourishing. Although more health is better than less, at least within a certain range, it is not the kind of good that can be maximized. No one aspires to be a virtuoso at health (except, perhaps, a hypochondriac). During the 1920s, eugenicists held health contests at state fairs and awarded prizes to the "fittest families." But this bizarre practice illustrates the folly of conceiving health in instrumental terms, or as a good to be maximized. Unlike the talents and traits that bring success in a competitive society, health is a bounded good; parents can seek it for their children without risk of being drawn into an ever-escalating arms race.

In caring for the health of their children, parents do not cast themselves as designers or convert their children into products of their will or instruments of their ambition. The same cannot be said of parents who pay large sums to select the sex of their child (for nonmedical reasons) or who aspire to bioengineer their child's intellectual endowments or athletic prowess. Like all distinctions, the line between therapy and enhancement blurs at the edges. (What about orthodontics, for example, or growth hormone for very short kids?) But this does not obscure the reason the distinction matters: parents bent on enhancing their children are more likely to overreach, to express and entrench attitudes at odds with the norm of unconditional love.

Of course, unconditional love does not require that parents refrain from shaping and directing the development of their child. To the contrary, parents have an obligation to cultivate their children, to help them discover and develop their talents and gifts. As May points out, parental love has two aspects: accepting love and transforming love. Accepting love affirms the being of the child, whereas transforming love seeks the well-being of the child. Each side of parental love corrects the excesses of the other: "Attachment becomes too quietistic if it slackens into mere acceptance of the child as he is." Parents have a duty to promote their child's excellence.

These days, however, overly ambitious parents are prone to get carried away with transforming love—promoting and demanding all manner of accomplishments from their children, seeking perfection. "Parents find it difficult to maintain an equilibrium between the two sides of love," May observes. "Accepting love, without transforming love, slides into indulgence and finally neglect. Transforming love, without accepting love, badgers and finally rejects." May finds in these competing impulses a parallel with modern science; it, too, engages us in beholding the given world, studying and savoring it, and also in molding the world, transforming and perfecting it.

The mandate to mold our children, to cultivate and improve them, complicates the case against enhancement. We admire parents who seek the best for their children, who spare no effort to help them achieve happiness and success. What, then, is the difference between providing such help through education and training and providing it by means of genetic enhancement? Some parents confer advantages on their children by enrolling, them in expensive schools, hiring private tutors, sending them to tennis camp, providing them with piano lessons, ballet lessons, swimming lessons, SAT prep courses, and so on. If it is permissible, even admirable, for parents to help their children in these ways, why isn't it equally admirable for parents to use whatever genetic technologies may emerge (provided they are safe) to enhance their child's intelligence, musical ability, or athletic skill?

Defenders of enhancement argue that there is no difference, in principle, between improving children through education and improving them through bioengineering. Critics of enhancement insist there is all the difference in the world. They argue that trying to improve children by manipulating their genetic makeup is reminiscent of eugenics, the discredited movement of the past century to improve the human race through policies (including forced sterilization and other odious measures) aimed at improving the gene pool. These competing analogies help clarify the moral status of genetic enhancement. Is the attempt of parents to enhance their children through genetic engineering more like education and training (a presumably good thing) or more like eugenics (a presumably bad thing)?

The defenders of enhancement are right to this extent: Improving children through genetic engineering is similar in spirit to the heavily managed, high-pressure child-rearing practices that have become common these days. But this similarity does not vindicate genetic enhancement. On the contrary, it highlights a problem with the trend toward hyperparenting. The most conspicuous examples are sports-crazed parents bent on making champions of their children. Sometimes they are successful, as in the case of Richard Williams, who reportedly planned the tennis careers of his daughters, Venus and Serena Williams, before they were born; or Earl Woods, who handed a golf club to young Tiger Woods while he was still in a playpen. "Let's face it, no kid puts themselves into a sport this way," Richard Williams told the *New York Times*. "The parents do it, and I'm guilty there. If you don't plan it, believe me, it's not going to happen."

A similar sentiment can be found outside the ranks of elite sports, among the overwrought parents on the sidelines of the soccer fields and Little League diamonds across the

Child Abuse in the Biotech Future

In the bioethic century, a parent's failure to correct genetic defects in utero might well be regarded as a heinous crime. Society may conclude that every parent has a responsibility to provide as safe and secure an environment as humanly possible for their unborn child. Not to do so might be considered a breach of parental duty for which the parents could be held morally, if not legally, liable. Mothers have already been held liable for having given birth to cocaine-addicted babies and babies with fetal alcohol syndrome. Prosecutors have argued that mothers passing on these painful addictions to their unborn children are culpable under existing child abuse statutes and ought to be held liable for the effect of their life style on their babies.

Proponents of human genetic engineering argue that it would be cruel and irresponsible not to use this powerful new technology to eliminate serious "genetic disorders." The problem with this argument, says the *New York Times* in an editorial entitled, "Whether to Make Perfect Humans," is that "there is no discernible line to be drawn between making inheritable repair of genetic defects and improving the species." The *Times* rightly points out that once scientist are able to repair genetic defects, "it will become much harder to argue against additional genes that confer desired qualities, like better health, looks, or brains."

Source Jeremy Rifkin,
Harvard International Review, *Spring 2005.*

land. So acute is the epidemic of parental intrusiveness and competitiveness that youth sports leagues have sought to control it by establishing parent-free zones, silent weekends (no yelling or cheering), and awards for parental sportsmanship and restraint.

Hectoring from the sidelines is not the only toll that hyperparenting takes on young athletes. As pickup games and playground sports have given way to sports leagues organized and managed by driving parents, pediatricians report an alarming increase in overuse injuries among teenagers. Today, sixteen-year-old pitchers are undergoing elbow reconstruction surgery, a procedure once performed only on major league pitchers seeking to prolong their careers. Dr. Lyle Micheli, the director of sports medicine at Boston Children's Hospital, reports that 70 percent of the young patients he treats suffer from overuse injuries, up from 10 percent twenty-five years ago. Sports doctors attribute the epidemic of overuse injuries to the growing tendency to have chidren specialize in a single sport from an early age, and to train for it year-round. "Parents think they are maximizing their child's chances by concentrating on one sport," said Dr. Micheli. "The results are often not what they expected."

Youth sports officials and doctors are not the only ones seeking ways to rein in overbearing parents. College administrators also complain of a growing problem with parents eager to control their children's lives—writing their children's college applications, phoning to badger the admissions office, helping write term papers, staying overnight in dorm rooms. Some parents even call college officials to ask that their child be awakened in the morning. "Parents of college students are out of control," says Marilee Jones, dean of admissions at MIT, who has made a mission or urging anxious parents to back off. Judith R. Shapiro, president of Barnard College, agrees. In an op-ed titled "Keeping Parents off Campus," she wrote: "Their sense of entitlement as consumers, along with an inability to let go, leads some parents to want to manage all aspects of their children's college lives—from the quest for admission to their choice of major. Such parents, while the exception, are nonetheless an increasing fact of life for faculty, deans and presidents." . . .

| *"Nature itself is indifferent to our dignity, and so altering nature cannot violate our dignity."*

Genetic Engineering Is Not Unethical

David Koepsell

In the following viewpoint, David Koepsell examines ethical objections to genetic engineering and finds most unconvincing. According to Koepsell, religious arguments that suggest genetic engineering is "playing God" fail to show how such experiments are not within a creator's plan or that a world without genetic engineering is preferred by such a creator. Addressing secular concerns about human dignity, Koepsell dismisses these by showing how genetic engineering can be used to aid sick individuals and keep them from suffering debilitating or terminal illness. Koepsell contends that humans have always intervened in the natural order to benefit themselves and that genetic engineering is merely another means to improve human life. David Koepsell is an author, philosopher, and attorney. He is the associate editor of Free Inquiry *and a professor of philosophy at the State University of New York at Buffalo.*

David Koepsell, "The Ethics of Genetic Engineering: A Position Paper from the Center for Inquiry, Office of Public Policy," Center for Inquiry, Office of Public Policy, August 2007. www.centerforinquiry.net. Reproduced by permission.

As you read, consider the following questions:

1. How does Koepsell refute the argument that genetic engineering is a misuse of human free will?

2. How does the author use the concept that "nature itself is indifferent to our dignity" to advance his argument?

3. Why is Koepsell not very concerned about the ethical arguments concerning genetic enhancement?

Just as the twentieth century was a golden age of computing, the twenty-first century is the DNA age. The silicon age brought about dramatic changes in how we as a species work, think, communicate, and play. The innovations of the computer revolution helped bring about the current genetic revolution, which promises to do for life what computing did for information. We are on the verge of being able to transform, manipulate, and create organisms for any number of productive purposes. From medicine, to agriculture, to construction and even computing, we are within reach of an age when manipulating the genetic codes of various organisms, or engineering entirely new organisms, promises to alter the way we relate to the natural world.

Biotechnology, specifically genetic engineering, is already a beneficial resource, employed in medicine, manufacturing, and agriculture. We have begun reaping the practical rewards of genetic engineering such as new medical therapies and increased crop yields and so far only a few instances of measurable harm have resulted. Genetic engineering has the potential to improve our health and well-being dramatically, revolutionize our manner of living, help us to conserve limited resources, and produce new wealth. Provided that it is appropriately regulated, bearing in mind ethical concerns relating to dignity, harmful consequences, and justice, its potential benefits outweigh its harms. There is certainly no reason to reject it outright as "unnatural." Biotechnology should be understood as an extension of already accepted and well-established techniques, such as directed breeding, combined with sophisticated understanding of evolution and genetic technologies.

As with any revolutionary technology, anxieties, fears, and moral objections to the promise of genetic engineering abound. Some are well-grounded and suggest caution, while others are the product of misinformation, religious prejudice, or hysteria. We should sort out those objections based on sound science and reason from those that are unfounded. Given the relative youth of the technology and the tremendous possibilities it offers for improvement of the human condition, as well as the environment in general, careful consideration of ethical implications now can help inform and ensure the future of the genetics era. . . .

Religious Objections Assume Too Much

Some people object to any tinkering with the genetic codes of humans, or even of any life form. Some religious critics perceive genetic engineering as "playing God" and object to it on the grounds that life is sacred and ought not to be altered by human intention. Other objectors argue from secular principles, such as the outspoken and ardent Jeremy Rifkin, who claims that it violates the inherent "dignity" of humans and other life-forms to alter their DNA under any circumstances. These arguments, while perhaps well-meaning, are not supported by sound logic or empirical evidence, as will be demonstrated here. Religious objections assume the existence of some creator whose will is defied by genetic engineering, and secular objections assume that life in its "natural" state, unaltered by human intention, is inviolable because of its inherent dignity.

Arguments based upon life's sacredness suggest that altering life forms violates the will of a creator, but they fail for want of internal theoretical consistency or because they rest on question-begging assumptions. If a creator does exist, most philosophers and theologians agree that either the creator's will is expressed in every facet of its creation, or that consistent with the creator's will mankind has free will, which includes the ability to create technologies. Thus, either genetic engineering can be seen as an expression of the creator's will—since it forms part of creation—or it is the result of our having been imbued with free will.

Granted, there are those who would claim that genetic engineering constitutes a misuse of our free will. Of course, determining what constitutes a misuse of our free will in defiance of divine directives depends on interpretation of those supposed divine directives. This is a problem with all moral theories premised on God's commands: what anyone believes to be commanded always depends on some human's interpretation of those commands. "Defying God's will" always means defying some person's interpretation of God's will. The difficulty of discerning a deity's wishes in the context of genetic engineering is compounded by the fact that none of the major religions' sacred writings speak to this issue. The Bible, for example, is silent on recombinant DNA. Furthermore, those who suggest that genetic engineering violates God's will must also view selective breeding of agricultural products, both plants and animals, as similarly contrary to God's will. If they do not view selective breeding as violating life's sacredness, then they must explain how it is qualitatively different from genetic engineering, which is in many ways only a quantitative or methodologically distinct process. The speed and predictability of the changes brought about by genetic engineering do surpass the speed and predictability of changes accomplished by selective breeding techniques, but that seems a poor argument for saying the former is contrary to God's will, while the latter is acceptable. Is it God's will that modifying nature is acceptable, but only provided we proceed slowly and haphazardly?

A Result of Inventiveness and Modification

Our entire culture exists by virtue of human inventiveness and our modification of nature. Even religious sects that reject modern technologies nonetheless embrace some technologies; the essence of technology is to alter the human relationship to nature. Clothing, agriculture, and weaponry have existed since before the dawn of civilization, and each alters our relationship with nature. These technologies express a rejection of the "natural" order of things, and result from human consciousness and intentionality. In fact, embracing these technologies has altered human evolution, enabling us to venture outside of the savannah, and live in a variety of climates, defending ourselves from inclement environments and dangerous predators. Without these technologies, it is likely that humans would look very different, with different strengths and weaknesses from those we see now, and would have remained in relatively restricted environments instead of populating six out of the seven continents (and the seventh to a limited extent). As such, the history of our tinkering with the natural is long, and its results generally lauded by religious and secular alike.

Technologies such as antibiotics and contraceptives have interfered with the natural order of evolution, preventing the conception of millions of human beings, and enabling the survival of others who might have died through exposure to diseases. These technologies have affected not only human populations, but also numerous species where humans have interfered through medicines, contraception, and selective breeding. Those who oppose the alteration of genomes of humans and other species based upon some notion of the inviolability of natural processes must provide an ethical justification of the use of medicines, contraception, and selective breeding which somehow sets them apart from conscious, more targeted alterations at the genetic level. The technical difference between genetic engineering and these other mechanisms of altering the natural evolution of various species is the difference between a blunderbuss and a rifle. The blunderbuss approach we have historically taken, by the use of contraception, antibiotics, and selective breeding, results in unanticipated consequences: medical and social problems may result from selecting for certain traits by breeding, or by ensuring the survival of potentially unfit members of the species through the use of medicines, or even by preventing generations of potentially fit members of a species being born. Moreover, these techniques are not always reliable in achieving their desired results. By contrast, genetic engineering is a rifle that can be accurately focused on a desired target. Admittedly, genetic engineering may have undesired side effects as well, but, as indicated, this does not distinguish this technique from currently accepted methods.

The Inherent Dignity Argument

Secular objectors to genetic engineering must defend the claim that the dignity of an individual member of a species, or of the species itself, is tied to its untampered-with evolution to its present state. This claim seems difficult to defend in light of the great infirmities—arguably indignities—that occur because of evolution, which is utterly indifferent to the suffering that results from many genetic disorders. Wholly innocent creatures lead lives of illness or degradation, or die prematurely because of genetic diseases. Where is the dignity in Lesch-Nyhan syndrome, a genetic disorder that results in uncontrollable self-mutilation? The dignity of individuals suffering from such infirmities is dependent not on their "natural" state, but on overcoming shortcomings or hardships.

Nature itself is indifferent to our dignity, and so altering nature cannot violate our dignity. In fact, it dignifies us to use the talents we have to alter our environment and our biology to improve our lives and those of the disabled. Technology in any form is an outgrowth of our intellectual abilities: at its best, it allows us to overcome natural shortcomings. Home heating and air conditioning violate the natural order, yet allow us to thrive in climates we otherwise could not survive. Few would argue that overcoming that natural disadvantage violates our inherent dignity.

Those who argue for drawing a line at altering the genome of humans or other organisms must give reasons both for regarding DNA as somehow special and apart from the rest of the natural world *and* for arguing that conscious manipulation of DNA is morally impermissible. There are some reasons to support "genetic exceptionalism," the point of view that DNA is unique, but those arguments do not necessarily imply: a) that because of this uniqueness there are absolute bars to altering it; or b) that if it is acceptable to alter the DNA of non-humans, it is nonetheless unacceptable to alter that of humans. Uniqueness does not itself imply any moral duty. In fact, every human being is "unique" by virtue of DNA, environment, and upbringing, but our moral duties toward each do not depend upon that uniqueness. Neither of the assumptions above can be sustained by logic or empirical evidence, and, as indicated previously, we have been tinkering with genes in plants, animals, and even human beings, through selective breeding for millennia. Thus, the uniqueness of DNA has never forbidden us implicitly or explicitly to modify what we encounter in nature.

Selective breeding can, over time, express genetic traits that are desired and suppress genes (and thus their phenotypes) that are undesired. Selective breeding manipulates the genome of a species, or subclasses of that species. As those who are familiar with various breeds of domesticated animals or plants, breeding for certain traits also has resulted in some instances in new and unanticipated infirmities. Genetic engineering allows for more selectivity in determining traits and in weeding out harmful traits or infirmities. It is arguably just a matter of degree rather than a qualitative difference in kind that separates selective breeding and genetic engineering. Those who oppose genetic engineering on moral grounds must make a coherent case that it is qualitatively different from selective breeding, or they must similarly oppose the selective breeding which has resulted in almost every aspect of our modern agriculture.

Compatible with Human Dignity

One of the problems in evaluating arguments based on "dignity" is in defining this concept. Many toss this word around without any explanation of its meaning. . . .

The concept of human dignity is perfectly compatible with genetic engineering. Recognizing human dignity often means taking steps to ensure that where nature impedes human potential, everyone's human potential may be achieved to the fullest. The disabled and the infirm should be aided wherever possible, and consistent with their stated goals, to achieve their potential, consistent with the principle of avoiding harm to others. Indeed, recognizing the inherent dignity of our fellow human beings suggests that we are impelled to pursue genetic engineering research, to the degree that it can help to develop therapies and treatments for those who suffer or develop natural or accidental limitations. Nor do enhancements pose an inherent threat to human dignity. Self-improvement is usually lauded, not condemned.

Clearly, some limits on genetic engineering also may be required by human dignity. Actions that diminish the capacities of others to achieve their potential are affronts to human dignity. Enslavement is the most extreme example, but less extreme diminutions to human dignity abound. Treating others as means to a personal end, for instance, rather than as an end in themselves diminishes the dignity of the one who is used, and impacts the dignity of the user. Genetic engineering requires special attention to issues of equal access and even some restrictions on its applications where they may threaten

A Utilitarian Defense

In the case of genetic engineering my broad assertion is that gene-technologies can, and probably will give people longer, healthier lives, with more choices and greater happiness. In fact, these technologies offer the possibility that we will be able to experience utilities greater and more intense than those on our current mental pallet. Genetic technology will bring advances in pharmaceuticals and the therapeutic treatment of disease, ameliorating many illnesses and forms of suffering. Somewhat further in the future our sense organs themselves may be re-engineered to allow us to perceive greater ranges of light and sound, our bodies re-engineered to permit us to engage in more strenuous activities, and our minds re-engineered to permit us to think more profound and intense thoughts. If utility is an ethical goal, direct control of our body and mind, through genetic control, cybernetics, prosthetics, or whatever, suggests the possibility of unlimited utility, and thus an immeasurable good.

J. Hughes,
Eubios Journal of Asian and International Bioethics,
June 1996.

subordination of some humans. Any invention used to diminish critical human capacities, such as cognitive functioning, would be unethical. Thus, while some people might benefit from a small race of humans genetically engineered to be slaves with diminished mental capacities this would clearly and egregiously violate human dignity. However, these objections effectively raise the issue of harms resulting from the misuse of genetic engineering, not the inherent immorality of genetic engineering. . . .

Benefits of Genetic Engineering

Genetic engineering has already supplied us with products that alleviate illness, clean up the environment, and increase crop yields, among other practical benefits to humanity and the ecosystem. For example, the first genetically engineered life form to be granted patent protection was developed by Ananda Chakrabarty, who genetically engineered a common bacterium into *Burkholderia cepacia*, a variant that digests petroleum products. He obtained a patent for his new life form, and helped establish the Supreme Court precedent that, to this day, enables inventors to patent genetically engineered life forms (*Diamond v. Chakrabarty* 1980). The bacterium cleans up oil spills and has proven to be both safe and useful. Since this precedent, tens of thousands of patents have been issued for genetically engineered life forms.

Genetic engineering has also helped create thousands of organisms and processes useful in medicine, research, and manufacturing. Genetically engineered bacteria churn out insulin for treating human diabetes, production of which would be substantially more expensive without the use of genetic engineering. The OncoMouse (U.S. Patent #75797027) was the first genetically engineered mouse to be patented for use as a model for cancer research. Numerous other "knock-out" mice have followed, each missing certain critical genes, or expressing certain genetic diseases, so that medical researchers can test drugs and other treatments for human genetic maladies without risking the lives of human subjects, and reducing the numbers of experimental animals sacrificed for science in the process. Gene therapy, in which manufactured viruses can deliver repairs to somatic cells with genetic defects, is making strides to correct genetic diseases or defects in fully grown humans.

Genetically engineered foods produce pest-resistant and drought-resistant crops, reducing the need for pesticides and fertilizers, and increasing yields in a world with an ever-growing need for food. Much of the so-called "green revolution" of the past few decades has been fueled by standard chemical technologies. New pesticides and remote sensing have enabled reductions in the amount of hazardous chemicals entering the ecosystem, and allowed farmers faced with an ever-expanding human population to meet the food needs of a planet. Nonetheless, insects and fungi, through evolutionary dynamics, develop resistance to pesticides. Moreover, even the best modern pesticides enter the food chain and the ecosystem, harming generations of humans and animals alike. Even in European countries like The Netherlands, farmers have recently had to switch from soil-growing plants to hydroponics due to the accumulation of toxic salts from fertilizers and pesticides. The promise of new genetic engineering technologies includes the development of pest-resistant strains of crops that would require little-to-no pesticides, or robust drought-resistant plants that can grow in harsh environments without irrigation.

Genetic engineering also holds the promise of creating new, more productive strains of farm animals for meat and milk production. These new strains may be more resistant to infections, reducing the need for large, unhealthy doses of antibiotics. They may also be engineered to produce more meat, so we need not slaughter as many animals, or they may produce milk or other products with vital nutrients otherwise not found in those products, ensuring a healthier source of such nutrients. Eventually, as envisioned in Margaret Atwood's *Oryx and Crake* (2003) [a dystopian novel on the consequences of globalization], animal variants used as food sources might even be engineered without anything more than an autonomous nervous system, arguably eradicating many of the ethical concerns involved with the wholesale slaughter of large mammals for food.

The Drawbacks

Of course, we need to assess our actions in light of both short and long-term consequences to the biosphere. Although the scientific consensus is that genetic engineering poses few, if any, short-term threats to the environment, long-term threats, known and unknown, must be considered as we move forward with research and genetic technologies. . . .

Somatic-cell and germline genetic engineering differ in important ways. Somatic cell therapy seeks to repair damage to cells that are not gametes [reproductive cells]. A creature with a genetic disease could theoretically be cured by somatic-cell therapy, and some advances have recently been made. One of the principal disadvantages of this process is its complexity. Repairing a fully grown organism means altering the genetic makeup of living cells.

Genetic engineering has made the most progress in germline alterations where the gametes of the organisms contain the altered DNA, and thus the organism's offspring carry the altered traits. This is the sort of engineering which has resulted in nearly every major scientific breakthrough and technological offshoot of genetic engineering. Altered bacteria, knock-out and other experimental animal models, and commercially available crops are among those that have resulted from germline genetic engineering.

Altering germ cells is a process that requires caution. Fertile organisms with altered germ cells may propagate beyond our control. This has happened with some genetically altered crops which have, in some instances, cross-fertilized non-engineered crops and spread their altered genes. This happened with Monsanto's "Terminator" corn, which renders its offspring infertile: farmers who chose not to use Monsanto's seeds nevertheless suffered the effects of infertile crops and could not use a portion of their crops to reseed because they had interbred with "Terminator" corn (U.S. Patent # 5723765, Control of Plant Expression). Seeds of neighboring non-genetically modified crops were "terminated" by cross-pollination, although the effects seem to have been limited to the first generation. . . .

How to Ensure Justice and Equality

Ethical principles and concerns about justice should act as a check on technological advancement. As distinct from science, which ought to be free to investigate any area of nature without restriction, technology brings scientific advancements that impact both humanity and the planetary environment for good or for ill. Apart from direct benefits or harms that may result from genetic engineering, which we have already considered, there is also the problem of how genetic engineering may affect the distribution of social goods as well as political rights. Such issues are often referred to as problems of distributive justice. . . .

With the onset of genetic engineering, there is a concern that genetic interventions, especially genetic enhancements—or the reverse, deliberate genetic disabling—may exacerbate already existing inequities as well as creating new ones. In evaluating these concerns, we need to bear in mind that genetic engineering is still young. Some of the possibilities discussed, such as creating new species of superhumans or subhumans, seem highly unlikely, at least for the foreseeable future. We are a long way from developing H.G. Wells-style Morlocks [subhuman worker-creatures from Wells's novel *The Time Machine*] to serve as our slaves. Nonetheless, although mad-scientist examples seem extreme, they are used by those who argue against the morality of using genetic engineering, and because many of these examples are within the range of technical possibility, they serve as useful illustrations for the underlying principles.

Beyond science-fiction examples, immediate issues involving access and social stratification impact on current notions of justice and should be worked out in public debate, perhaps legislation. As with any new and expensive medical technology, non-socialized medical regimes in which genetic interventions become available will likely result in stratification of services and beneficiaries. There will be the class of those who can afford access to new technologies, and those who cannot. This will not be a unique situation, for already a number of elective and even necessary medical procedures are unavailable to the segment of the population that cannot afford them, or has inadequate or no health insurance. Inequality of access raises obvious social justice concerns where treatments or services are medically necessary which might not be available to everyone because of cost.

As with cosmetic enhancements presently available, genetic enhancements threaten to create a class division between the "haves" and "have-nots." Even now, cosmetic surgery confers some tangible economic and social benefits on those who can afford it. While a genetic underclass of slaves seems far-fetched, consider, for instance, parents who decide they want their child to be an NBA (National Basketball Association) player, so they select for traits conferring height, stamina and intense athleticism. Such a genetically enhanced individual will enjoy benefits that no amount of training could provide for the most motivated, unenhanced person. In such a possible future, one of the means by which poor yet motivated people now move from an underclass position to one of economic security may well disappear, given unfair competition from players whose parents could afford genetic enhancement. Similar scenarios can be envisioned for a range of abilities, including intelligence, musical ability, physical attractiveness, etc.

Although possession of these traits now confers some social and economic advantage, it is now the result of chance and evolution (which is largely unpredictable). In a world where genetic enhancement is available but not readily affordable, only the rich will be able to stack the deck in favor of their children.

Of course we face similar social-ethical issues with other technologies, but in the realm of genetic modification, decisions are more complex. Cosmetic enhancements are not heritable, but the possibility of a new genetic aristocracy is both technically feasible and troubling. However, we must also recognize that it will be difficult to coordinate and establish rational oversight and regulation of germline modifications in humans while respecting both autonomy and the need to guard against social injustice. There is a presumption that self-improvement is permissible, if not laudable, even when it provides someone with a competitive advantage for herself and her offspring. We would regard as unacceptable legislation prohibiting someone from going to law school or medical school merely because she comes from a wealthy family and can easily afford the tuition. If use of one's money for a superior education is permissible, can we confidently say that use of one's money to alter one's genes to obtain a higher IQ for oneself and one's offspring is impermissible? For now, the technology is nowhere near marketable, so we have time for a clearheaded dialogue about the social justice issues associated with genetic modification by choice.

> *"We believe that . . . attempts to produce a cloned child would be highly unethical."*

Human Cloning is Unethical

President's Council on Bioethics

The President's Council on Bioethics is a commission of experts appointed directly by the president of the United States that advises him on ethical issues related to advances in biomedical science and technology. The following viewpoint is the council's report to the president on the issue of human cloning. The council contends that "cloning-to-produce-children" is wholly unethical in terms of both research and humanity. They argue that cloned children will experience problems of identity and individuality and troubled family relations, among other things. The council also believes cloning will ultimately alter society for the worse.

As you read, consider the following questions:

1. What is a major weakness in the arguments supporting cloning-to-produce-children, according to this study?
2. What are the ethical principles that should guide a broader assessment of cloning-to-produce-children, according to the Council?

The President's Council on Bioethics, "Human Cloning and Human Dignity: An Ethical Inquiry," July 2002. www.bioethics.gov.

3. What are the five categories of concern that the Council has identified regarding cloning-to-produce-children?

The prospect of human cloning has been the subject of considerable public attention and sharp moral debate, both in the United States and around the world. Since the announcement in February 1997 of the first successful cloning of a mammal (Dolly the sheep), several other species of mammals have been cloned. Although a cloned human child has yet to be born, and although the animal experiments have had low rates of success, the production of functioning mammalian cloned offspring suggests that the eventual cloning of humans must be considered a serious possibility. . . .

The Debate over Human Cloning

The debate over human cloning became further complicated in 1998 when researchers were able, for the first time, to isolate human embryonic stem cells. Many scientists believe that these versatile cells, capable of becoming any type of cell in the body, hold great promise for understanding and treating many chronic diseases and conditions. Some scientists also believe that stem cells derived from *cloned* human embryos, produced explicitly for such research, might prove uniquely useful for studying many genetic diseases and devising novel therapies. . . .

What Is at Stake?

The intense attention given to human cloning in both its potential uses, for reproduction as well as for research, strongly suggests that people do not regard it as just another new technology. Instead, we see it as something quite different, something that touches fundamental aspects of our humanity. The notion of cloning raises issues about identity and individuality, the meaning of having children, the difference between procreation and manufacture, and the relationship between the generations. It also raises new questions about the manipulation of some human beings for the benefit of others, the freedom and value of biomedical inquiry, our obligation to heal the sick (and its limits), and the respect and protection owed to nascent human life.

Finally, the legislative debates over human cloning raise large questions about the relationship between science and society, especially about whether society can or should exercise ethical and prudential control over biomedical technology and the conduct of biomedical research. Rarely has such a seemingly small innovation raised such big questions. . . .

The Ethics of Cloning-to-Produce Children

Two separate national-level reports on human cloning concluded that attempts to clone a human being would be unethical at this time due to safety concerns and the likelihood of harm to those involved. The Council concurs in this conclusion. But we have extended the work of these distinguished bodies by undertaking a broad ethical examination of the merits of, and difficulties with, cloning-to-produce-children.

Cloning-to-produce-children might serve several purposes. It might allow infertile couples or others to have genetically-related children; permit couples at risk of conceiving a child with a genetic disease to avoid having an afflicted child; allow the bearing of a child who could become an ideal transplant donor for a particular patient in need; enable a parent to keep a living connection with a dead or dying child or spouse; or enable individuals or society to try to "replicate" individuals of great talent or beauty. These purposes have been defended by appeals to the goods of freedom, existence (as opposed to nonexistence), and well-being—all vitally important ideals.

A major weakness in these arguments supporting cloning-to-produce-children is that they overemphasize the freedom, desires, and control of parents, and pay insufficient attention to the well-being of the cloned child-to-be. The Council holds that, once the child-to-be is carefully considered, these arguments are not sufficient to overcome the powerful case against engaging in cloning-to-produce-children.

First, cloning-to-produce-children would violate the principles of the ethics of human research. Given the high rates of morbidity and mortality in the cloning of other mammals, we believe that cloning-to-produce-children would be extremely unsafe, and that attempts to produce a cloned child would be highly unethical. Indeed, our moral analysis of this matter leads us to conclude that this is not, as is sometimes implied, a merely temporary objection, easily removed by the improvement of technique. We offer arguments in support of a strong conclusion: that conducting experiments in an effort to make cloning-to-produce-children less dangerous would itself be an unacceptable violation of the norms of research ethics. *There seems to be no ethical way to try to discover whether cloning-to-produce-children can become safe, now or in the future.*

Categories of Concern

If carefully considered, the concerns about safety also begin to reveal the ethical principles that should guide a broader assessment of cloning-to-produce-children: the principles of freedom, equality, and human dignity. To appreciate the broader human significance of cloning-to-produce-children, one needs first to reflect on the meaning of having children; the meaning of asexual, as opposed to sexual, reproduction; the importance of origins and genetic endowment for identity and sense of self; the meaning of exercising greater human control over the processes and "products" of human reproduction; and the difference between begetting and making. Reflecting on these topics, the Council has identified five categories of concern regarding cloning-to-produce-children. (Different Council Members give varying moral weight to these different concerns.)

The Question of Informed Consent

Too often ... risks are dismissed in the name of informed consent, the duty to disclose and warn patients or research participants of risks to their health and well-being. The argument is that if women are informed about the risks of egg extraction for research, it should be their choice as to whether they assume those risks and provide their eggs.

However, it is not entirely accurate to speak of "informed consent" when there is a lack of independent assessment about the long-term health risks of egg harvesting. As [K.K.] Ahuja *et al.*, remark, "[The] present uncertainty and the paucity of meaningful statistics diluted 'informed consent'". However, some research links egg harvesting to hormonal cancers. Scientific investigation of these long-term risks is required before women can meaningfully consent to egg extraction for research....

[Additionally], consent does not occur within a vacuum, but always within a context. Women's decisions to provide ova should be considered against the background of powerful social and economic forces that have vested interests in women's decisions about their eggs: the biotechnology industry, scientists, research advocates and patients themselves who may well exercise influence—albeit well meaning—in the hope of treatments.

As [D.] Beeson and [A.] Lippman have noted, some physicians who extract eggs are also involved in cloning research. "Seeking consent from women in these circumstances is problematic when clinicians have an interest in obtaining their eggs". This is not to assert that women are incapable of exercising choice in this context. But it does require us to question the value, worth and power of a woman's decision to provide ova.

Katrina George, Reproductive BioMedicine Online, *August 2007. www.rbmonline.com.*

- *Problems of identity and individuality.* Cloned children may experience serious problems of identity both because each will be genetically virtually identical to a human being who has already lived and because the expectations for their lives may be shadowed by constant comparisons to the life of the "original."

- *Concerns regarding manufacture.* Cloned children would be the first human beings whose entire genetic makeup is selected in advance. They might come to be considered more like products of a designed manufacturing process than "gifts" whom their parents are prepared to accept as they are. Such an attitude toward children could also contribute to increased commercialization and industrialization of human procreation.

- *The prospect of a new eugenics.* Cloning, if successful, might serve the ends of privately pursued eugenic enhancement, either by avoiding the genetic defects that may arise when human reproduction is left to chance, or by preserving and perpetuating outstanding genetic traits, including the possibility, someday in the future, of using cloning to perpetuate genetically engineered enhancements.

- *Troubled family relations.* By confounding and transgressing the natural boundaries between generations, cloning could strain the social ties between them. Fathers could become "twin brothers" to their "sons"; mothers could give birth to their genetic twins; and grandparents would also be the "genetic parents" of their grandchildren. Genetic relation to only one parent might produce special difficulties for family life.

- *Effects on society.* Cloning-to-produce-children would affect not only the direct participants but also the entire society that allows or supports this activity. Even if practiced on a small scale, it could affect the way society looks at children and set a precedent for future nontherapeutic interventions into the human genetic endowment or novel forms of control by one generation over the next. In the absence of wisdom regarding these matters, prudence dictates caution and restraint.

Conclusion: For some or all of these reasons, the Council is in full agreement that cloning-to-produce-children is not only unsafe but also morally unacceptable, and ought not to be attempted.

> "The actual opposition to human clon-
> ing springs from something primordial,
> the fear of the unknown, the fear cap-
> tured in the catch-phrase: 'We can't
> play God.' But why can't we?"

Human Cloning Is Not Unethical

Harry Binswanger

*In the following viewpoint, Harry Binswanger contends that hu-
man cloning should not be banned. Binswanger argues that humans have always excelled at overcoming nature's limitations to
improve individual lives and the lot of society. He insists that
cloning is just another instance of humans using their intelligence to make scientific breakthroughs. To thwart such experiments, he believes, is tantamount to sacrificing human lives to
unjustifiable fears. For this reason, he sees a ban on cloning as
morally wrong. Harry Binswanger is a professor of philosophy at
the Objectivist Academic Center of the Ayn Rand Institute in
California.*

As you read, consider the following questions:

1. Why does Binswanger believe no one's rights would be
   violated by human cloning?

Harry Binswanger, "Immoral to Ban Human Cloning: Irrational Fears Must Not Block Scientific Advances," *Capitalism Magazine*, December 19, 2003. www.capmag.com. Reproduced by permission.

2. What makes up a person's essential self, according to the author?

3. Apart from the issue of cloning, how does the human race already "play God," in Binswanger's view?

On [July 30, 2001], the [George W.] Bush administration declared itself "unequivocally opposed" to human cloning, whether for stem-cell research or reproduction. "The moral and ethical issues posed by human cloning are profound and cannot be ignored in the quest for scientific discovery."

The premise here is apparent: until a scientist can satisfy the religiously minded, the scientist cannot proceed. Science functions by permission of religion. On this premise, we would not have anesthesia, birth control, or, arguably, the wheel.

In a free society, the principle is not: ban everything, then allow a few exceptions. Rather, the government cannot ban anything except acts that violate individual rights.

But whose rights would be violated by human cloning?

If the cloning is used for research, the product is a microscopic group of cells. One could argue about the status of a fetus in the late stages of pregnancy, but there are no rational grounds for ascribing rights to a clump of cells in a Petri dish.

If the cloning is used for reproduction, the result is a baby who exactly resembles, physically, someone else. Again, whose rights would that violate? If no one's, what is the justification for government even to consider stepping in to ban it?

If you were cloned today, nine months from now a woman would give birth to a baby with your genetic endowment. The cloned baby would be your identical twin, delayed a generation.

Twins of the same age do not frighten us, so why should a twin separated by a generation?

Some fear the specter of mass cloning of one individual, especially cloning of sadistic monsters, as in *The Boys from*

Brazil, Ira Levin's nightmarish projection of cadres of young Hitlers spawned from the dictator's genes.

The error here is philosophical: equating a person with his body. A person's essential self is his mind—that in him which thinks, values, and chooses. It is one's mind, not one's genes, that governs who one is. Man is the rational animal. One's basic choice is to think or not to think, in Ayn Rand's phrase, and the conclusions, values, and character of individuals depend upon the extent and rationality of their thinking.

Genes provide the capacity to reason, but the exercise and guidance of that capacity is up to each individual, from the birth of his reasoning mind in infancy through the rest of his life.

Neither genes nor environment can implant ideas in a child's mind and make him accept them. Only his own self-generated thinking—or his default on that responsibility—will shape his soul.

Cloning the body will not clone the mind. A mind is inescapably under the individual's own volitional control. *The Boys from Brazil*? It was not Hitler's body but his choices that made him a monster.

The worry about this kind of problem cannot account for the virtual panic over human cloning, nor for the fact that the anti-cloning clique opposes human cloning across the board, in any quantity, for any reason.

The actual opposition to human cloning springs from something primordial, the fear of the unknown, the fear captured in the catch-phrase: "We can't play God." But why can't we? We can and we must.

A surgeon "plays God" whenever he removes a cancer or an infected appendix rather than letting the patient die. We "play God" anytime we use our intelligence to improve the "natural" course of events. Natural? It is man's nature to "play God" by reshaping matter to produce the food, shelter, tools, cars, and power stations that sustain and enhance our exist-

Cloning Is Not Immoral—
Bad Parenting Is

Some opponents of cloning believe that such individuals would be wronged in morally significant ways. Many of these wrongs involve the denial of what [political and social philospher] Joel Feinberg has called "the right to an open future." For example, a child might be constantly compared to the adult from whom he was cloned, and thereby burdened with oppressive expectations. Even worse, the parents might actually limit the child's opportunities for growth and development. . . . Finally, regardless of his parents' conduct or attitudes, a child might be burdened by the *thought* that he is a copy and not an "original." The child's sense of self-worth or individuality or dignity, so some have argued, would thus be difficult to sustain.

How should we respond to these concerns? On the one hand, the existence of a right to an open future has a strong intuitive appeal. We are troubled by parents who radically constrict their children's possibilities for growth and development. Obviously, we would condemn a cloning parent for crushing a child with oppressive expectations, just as we might condemn fundamentalist parents for utterly isolating their children from the modern world, or the parents of twins for inflicting matching wardrobes and rhyming names. But this is not enough to sustain an objection to cloning itself. Unless the claim is that cloning parents cannot help but be oppressive, we would have cause to say they had wronged their children only because of their subsequent, and avoidable, sins of bad parenting—not because they had chosen to create the child in the first place.

Robert Wachbroit,
Report from the Institute for Philosphy & Public Policy,
Fall 1997.

ence. Not to "play God" in this way means to abandon the struggle for human life and submit uncomplainingly to whatever happens.

Stem-cell research holds the promise of major breakthroughs in saving actual human lives—yours and mine. The potential human being that could, in principle, be produced from the cells in that Petri dish is just that: a potential person, not an actual one. The idea of banning such research to sacrifice actual lives to potential ones is wrong morally and politically.

At the threshold of a wide range of earth-shaking biomedical advances, we must not let irrational fears of the new slow progress in the battle to enhance and extend human life.

"When a genetically modified seed is able to replicate and carry its features on to the next generation of consumers, it poses special ethical issues."

Genetically Engineered Food Poses Ethical Concerns

Britt Bailey

In the following viewpoint, Britt Bailey poses concerns about the possible harms of genetically engineered (GE) food. Asserting that the safety of such food has not been proven, Bailey suggests that problems, such as allergic reactions to GE food, might fall hardest on children and other susceptible people. Bailey also claims that biotech food might be less nutritious than organic food—a considerable dilemma considering genetically engineered foods were designed in part to help feed the malnourished. Bailey states that because of the unknowns associated with biotech food, their use could be unethical, especially if potential problems severely impacted vulnerable populations. Britt Bailey is the founder and director of Environmental Commons, a public edu-

Britt Bailey, "Can Genetically Engineered Foods Compromise Social Equality?" EnvironmentalCommons, 1999. www.environmentalcommons.org. Reproduced by permission.

cation and advocacy organization promoting conservation and environmental protection. She is the coauthor of Against the Grain: Biotechnology and the Corporate Takeover of Your Food.

As you read, consider the following questions:

1. According to Bailey, what percentage of foods in the United States contain some genetically engineered components or by-products?
2. Food allergens are usually contained in what type of organic compound, according to the author?
3. As Bailey states it, what is the ethical notion of equivalency?

Both the volume and extent of genetically altered food crops newly introduced into our food supply ensures they will have an impact on society. New genetic sequences are often introduced into such food crops from disparate species assuring a de minimus [trivial] deviation from conventional food products. Of necessity, when a genetically modified seed is able to replicate and carry its features on to the next generation of consumers, it poses special ethical issues both now and in the future. The central public health and ethical questions center on whether engineered changes are sufficiently new enough to pose unanticipated health risks, and if so, do they impact differentially on varying members of the population.

If genetically engineered foods differ significantly in terms of adverse health impacts, the skewed distribution could disproportionately burden vulnerable populations, exacerbating health gaps already created by differential access to health care and exposure to toxic substances. For instance, persons with deficient metabolizing or detoxifying systems including children may be unjustly burdened by genetically engineered foods. Some infants and newborns, especially those living in poorer socioeconomic conditions, may have little or no choice but to eat genetically engineered foods. This is because their parents' food choices are constrained by poverty or because non-genetically engineered (e.g., organic) foods are unavailable.

Disadvantaged or Vulnerable Populations

Currently in the United States, no mandate exists to label genetically engineered foods, in spite of the fact that 65–75% of the foods sold contain genetically engineered components or byproducts in the form of new proteins. This reality conflicts with consumers' legitimate desires for labels that would reveal the presence of byproducts of genetic modification in their food. Presently the only way to avoid genetically engineered foods is by purchasing organic foods, which by definition exclude genetically modified material. But many families are unable to purchase such premium price, non-genetically engineered goods, raising the question of access to non-genetically engineered foods. More critically, should any novel protein adversely stimulate the immune system, the inability of persons in the lower socioeconomic strata (for whom asthma and food allergies are special problems) to avoid such foods raises a critical question of the equitable distribution of risk in society.

A second issue hinges on whether or not genetically engineered foods are in any way nutritionally deficient or defective compared to their conventional counterparts. Our own work suggests soybeans may lose valuable phytoestrogens after being genetically engineered. (We have recently confirmed our initial finding of below conventional levels—by some 12–18%—of genistin and daidzin in a third series of tests). Were genetically engineered foods, which are presently flooding world markets at below par prices, to prove nutritionally inferior as a group, they could compromise the very populations the life-science industry claims to be interested in aiding.

Special Attention to Children

The fact that children seem to be more likely to react adversely to novel foods than do adults makes it important to ask if genetically engineered foods pose any undue burden upon this young population. Foods derived from the advances in genetic technology include new and potentially allergenic proteins coded by their novel genotypes. Should children from lower socioeconomic strata experience an especially elevated risk, such as from allergic reactions, as a result of their increased exposure to genetically engineered antigens, the inability of their parents to "exit" the system (e.g. no labels; because of the high price of organic foods, limited availability of conventional foods, etc.) compounds the ethical problem.

The debate surrounding the alteration of the food supply, has been entrusted to the science community with very little input from those with differing philosophical and perceptual convictions. For instance, the scientific community has continued to debate the equivalency of genetically engineered foods in relationship to conventionally created ones, while neglecting the potential secondary effects of novel foodstuffs on exposed populations, or the necessity to perform extensive safety testing to assure the well-being of infants or children.

In spite of only a tiny fraction of the necessary testing being completed, the Food and Drug Administration has declared foods derived via molecular biology to be analogous to conventionally bred foods. Likewise the life-science industry has published data asserting the comparability of genetically engineered foods, and have even claimed the novel foods may improve health and nutrition. However, the novel genes and their products, many originating from bacteria, have not been tested adequately for long-term safety. Nor have the food's active biological chemicals been tested for significant alterations which might create novel antigenic configurations, e.g. through differential folding of genetically engineered proteins.

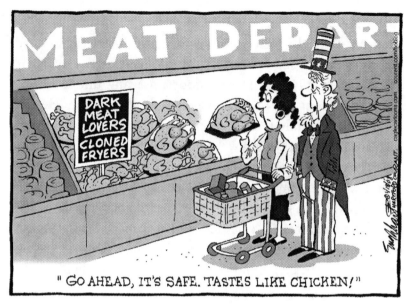

" GO AHEAD, IT'S SAFE. TASTES LIKE CHICKEN! "

© 2008 Bob Englehart, *The Hartford Courant*, and PoliticalCartoons.com.

Allergenicity

These realities are particularly eventful in light of the potential allergenicity posed by new genes which program for novel proteins. In part because of this concern, the National Academy of Sciences, after thorough review of potential harms stemming from genetically engineered crops, has recommended an extended testing protocol for allergenicity.

Allergenic reactions can cause discomfort, including shortness of breath, hives, and in some cases can cause life-threatening anaphylactic shock. Since known food allergens tend to be proteins, foods with new proteins added via genetic engineering could potentially become newly allergenic food sources. Eighty-eight percent of people suffering from food allergies are "atopic" in that they have other allergic reactions, including asthma or rhinitis, an inflammation of the nasal mucous membrane causing a runny nose and sneezing.

Were allergenicity to prove to be a problem, it would almost certainly impact differentially on the poor, and affect children specifically. Food allergies tend to affect susceptible individuals. They have become a serious public health concern, affecting roughly 2.5 to 5 million Americans. Up to two million, or 8%, of children in the U.S. are affected by food allergies as are up to 2% of adults. Food allergens—those parts of foods that cause allergic reactions—are usually proteins. Many food allergens can still cause reactions even after they are cooked or have resisted the degradation which normally accompanies digestion. Some like the Cry 1A toxins expressed in insect resistant genetically engineered plants (for human consumption) fit this latter category.

Most proteins added to foods via genetic engineering cannot be tested directly for allergenicity prior to their incorporation into a foodstuff. Instead, industry scientists simply screen the biochemical characteristics of proteins to see if they are "consistent" with the characteristics associated with allergens. It remains to be seen how effective such screening will be in protecting the health of vulnerable populations of the public.

The Ethical Question of Equality

In order to decide that special duty of care is owed to children who may be placed at a greater disadvantage due to the marketing and ubiquitous nature of genetically modified foods, there needs first to be a discussion as to why society should give special consideration to susceptible populations. The underlying premise for such consideration is the notion of equivalency: if two groups with varying degrees of vulnerability to a health limiting factor are to be kept equal in health outcome, the more vulnerable group requires differential treatment. In its broad sense, justice requires that distribution be fair as a means of respecting the equality of deservedness under an equal rights doctrine or to assure the fair distribution of goods in a system designed to guarantee equality of outcomes and/or utility.

Recall that as an independent ethical principle, justice permits a pattern of distribution to be morally right even if it conflicts with maximizing the aggregate social good. When patterns of distribution or risk status are unequal, such as when one group is disproportionately burdened with a health risk, egalitarian justice would defend assistance to those worse off.

Recall also that egalitarian theory strives for an equality of well-being, not of sameness. In the circumstance of the distribution of genetically engineered foods, the relevant question is whether children generally, and the children of adults not having access to non-genetically foods specifically, have equal opportunity to achieve well-being as do those with the means to avoid potentially deficient harmful foods. This problem is exacerbated if genetically engineered foods create differential risks, say by virtue of their allergenicity, nutritional composition, or specific deficiencies, thereby unjustly burdening susceptible populations. Conversely, preferential marketing protections and "streamlined" safety testing might be justified if enhanced gene products had greater nutritional levels, greater yields, etc. Were these advantages afforded to "higher quality" genetically engineered foods under this system, it could be justified under the principle whereby basic inequalities are justified only when they work to the advantage of the socially worst-off group.

Genetically engineered foods thus may not deserve their apparent preferential treatment if they are not in fact "better." If the foods do place children and in particular children from lower socioeconomic classes at an increased rate of risk for allergenic reactions they would be deserving of differential restrictions, not permissiveness. What is clear is that no one has determined whether or not genetically engineered foods are physiologically neutral, inferior, or better than conventional varieties already on the market. Given that the new genetically engineered varieties have virtually supplanted their predecessors, the ethical question of equality is central to a deliberation of value to vulnerable populations. The penultimate question turns on whether we are permitting the creation of foods which could place an already vulnerable population at potentially greater risk instead of creating foods and new technologies which could truly create better health particularly for those who are worse off.

Periodical Bibliography

The following articles have been selected to supplement the diverse views presented in this chapter.

Anita L. Allen	"Genetic, and Moral, Enhancement," *Chronicle of Higher Education*, May 16, 2008.
Nick Bostrom	"In Defense of Posthuman Dignity," *Bioethics*, June 2005.
Richard Brookhiser	"Matters of Morality," *Time*, August 6, 2007.
Sholto Byrnes	"There Is a Debate to Be Had—a Serious Debate—About Conscience," *New Statesman*, May 26, 2008.
Christianity Today	"The Slope Really Is Slippery," March 2007.
Freeman Dyson	"Our Biotech Future," *New York Review of Books*, July 19, 2007.
Ronald M. Green	"Are Babies by Design in Our Future?" *Personalized Medicine*, August 2008.
Richard Hayes	"Our Biopolitical Future," *World Watch*, March/April 2007.
Cindy Kuzma	"Of Manimals and Humanzees," *Science & Spirit*, November/December 2006.
S. Matthew Liao	"The Ethics of Using Genetic Engineering for Sex Selection," *Journal of Medical Ethics*, February 2005.
Mark Lynas	"We Must Stop Trying to Engineer Nature," *New Statesman*, February 26, 2007.
Bruno Maddox	"Who's Freaky Now?" *Discover*, October 2006.
Robin McKie	"Religion Must Not Block Progress," *New Statesman*, May 19, 2008.
Patrick Tucker	"Genetic Ethics and 'Superbabies,'" *Futurist*, January/February 2008.

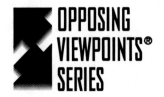

CHAPTER 3

What Is the Impact of Genetically Engineered Foods?

Chapter Preface

In 2007, the United States Department of Agriculture (USDA) and the Animal and Plant Inspection Service (APIS) deregulated the growing of genetically engineered (GE), herbicide-resistant sugar beets and allowed for their growth and distribution on a commercial scale. These modified sugar beet seeds have been engineered to withstand the widely used herbicide brand Round-Up in an attempt to control weed populations in sugar beet crops while maintaining plant health. However, since the USDA and the APIS approved the widespread use of these GE seeds, their use has stirred controversy and debate.

On January 23, 2008, the Center for Food Safety, along with the Organic Seed Alliance, the Sierra Club, and High Mowing Organic Seeds, filed a lawsuit against both federal entities citing the environmental impacts that Round-Up-resistant sugar beets would cause. Wind-blown pollen from genetically engineered crops could contaminate conventionally and organically grown vegetables—a detriment to farmers and consumers alike, these organizations claim. The groups also contend that the use of herbicides would be increased because it would allow farmers to use chemicals without fear of damaging the beet crops. Studies have also shown that the second generation of Round-Up-resistant seeds are twice as resistant as their parents, increasing fears of indiscriminate herbicide use. The biggest concern is the potential spread of glyphosate, the chief ingredient in Round-Up and other herbicides. Glyphosate is acutely toxic to humans; less than a cupful (237ml) is lethal. The widespread use of such toxins could prove dangerous to people, as well as to such beneficial creatures as lacewings, predatory mites, ladybugs, and earthworms.

Furthermore, independent analysis of USDA data done by Dr. Charles Benbrook, former board of agriculture chair of the National Academy of Sciences, showed that in 2006, 81 percent of genetically engineered crops were those that had been modified to be herbicide resistant and that 99 percent of those grown in the United States were "Round-Up resistant" plants. According to Benbrook, the growth of these GE plants increased herbicide use by 122 pounds, a fifteenfold increase, in the ten years that genetically engineered crops had been grown in the United States.

Companies such as American Crystal Sugar and Kellogg's have come out in support of the genetically engineered sugar beets. American Crystal Sugar, America's largest sugar beet processor, plans to use the modified beets, and Kellogg's spokeswoman Kris Charles said her company "would not have any issues" buying sugar from genetically engineered beets.

In the following chapter, other advocates and detractors of genetically engineered food and livestock debate whether these innovations should raise hopes about increased food production or increase fears about safety and environmental impact.

"There are, actually, many facts that support the safeness of biotech food."

Genetically Modified Foods Are Safe

Karri Hammerstrom

In the following viewpoint, Karri Hammerstrom contends that farmers should utilize biotechnology and genetic engineering to increase the safety and productivity of their crops. She rebuts numerous complaints leveled against the use and proliferation of genetically modified (GM) crops and argues that organic farming, often offered as a safe and environmentally friendly alternative to GM crops, does not actually provide any benefits over GM crops. Karri Hammerstrom is a member of the Environmental Protection Agency's Farm, Ranches, and Rural Communities Advisory Committee, and she farms peaches, plums, and alfalfa in the San Joaquin Valley in California.

As you read, consider the following questions:

1. According to Hammerstrom, what is the cost and length of time needed for testing a genetically modified (GM) plant before it becomes available to consumers?

Karri Hammerstrom, "The Future of Food and Medicine," *AgBioWorld*, September 2005. www.agbioworld.org. Reproduced by permission.

2. According to studies cited by the author, how are the production of crops, farm income, use of pesticides, and prevalence of pesticide poisonings affected when GM crops are used by farmers?

3. In addition to claims that GM crops are unsafe, what are some of the other unsubstantiated myths about GM crops that Hammerstrom attempts to debunk?

As a mother and a consumer, I want to know that the food I eat and prepare for my family is safe and nutritious. I also want to know that technological advances are occurring to keep the food safe. . . .

I have spent many hours educating myself on the pros and cons of biotechnology and genetically modified foods. I have read numerous articles, searched the internet, listened to renowned experts on the subject, and talked to friends and family regarding biotechnology, which is the refinement of conventional breeding of plants and animals to achieve desired, beneficial traits. I have also tried desperately to understand what, in my opinion, are the misguided and unjustified fears of those vehemently opposed to biotechnology. My conclusion is that rather than having opposition based on reality or fact, that those opposed, or posing as the opposition, truly just dislike the United States' government (which ironically allows them to freely have an opposing view), successful multinational corporations, and anything that flies in the face of their organic dogma which really has very little to do with organic farming.

The Job of the Family Farmer

After watching *The Future of Food* (an anti-biotech film), I was deeply troubled by the irresponsible pseudo-documentary which tries to present lies as truth and fiction as fact. While trying to unabashedly espouse their anti-government and anti-multinational corporate sentiment, the anti-biotechnology activists responsible for the film take an unjustified swing at the family farmer who chooses to farm conventionally and who may choose to incorporate biotechnology into their operations.

That is where I saw *The Future of Food* crossing the line. You see, in addition to being a mother and a consumer, I am also a farmer. I consider myself and my peers to be environmental stewards of the land, as well as farmland preservationists. Like 99 percent of all U.S. farms, my farm is family owned and operated. In fact, according to the 2002 Census of Agriculture only less than 1 percent of America's farms and ranches are owned by non-family corporations. And, about 94 percent of U.S. agricultural products sold are produced on farms like mine that are owned by individuals, family partnerships and family corporations. Non-family corporations account for only about 6 percent of U.S. agricultural product sales.

In spite of burdensome regulations and increased urbanization, California is still the number one agricultural producer and exporter in the United States. Contributing almost $30 billion to the economy, California farmers raise more than 350 different crops that supply food, fiber and flowers to the world. California agriculture also supports over 1.1 million jobs or nearly 8 percent of all the jobs in the state. Farming is by no means an easy profession, but it is a noble one and I am proud of what I do and how I do it.

The film noted above tries to invoke hysteria into the biotechnologically-challenged masses (i.e. the average consumer, like me, who wants a variety of convenient, healthful foods at reasonable costs, but otherwise does not want to be troubled with the details) by conveying that conventional farming involving biotechnology is dangerous and that organic farming is the purest farming above all others. There are, actually, many facts that support the safeness of biotech food. Here are a few:

A History of Genetically Modified Foods

First, conventional farming and the use of biotechnology are safe. For centuries, humankind has made improvements to plants through selective breeding and hybridization—the controlled pollination of plants. Plant biotechnology is an extension of traditional plant breeding with one very important difference—biotechnology ensures the transfer of beneficial traits in a precise, controlled manner. Crops developed through biotechnology are subject to testing and monitoring at three levels of the federal government which secure food and environmental safety of biotechnology derived products. Specifically, the U.S. Department of Agriculture (USDA) makes sure the products are safe to grow; the U.S. Food and Drug Administration (FDA) makes sure the products are safe to eat; and the U.S. Environmental Protection Agency (EPA) regulates crop protection characteristics.

Critics of biotechnology have claimed that some crops are not tested and pandemonium may occur by growing unchecked crops. The emergence of a new genetically modified plant variety on the market is not the beginning, but the end result of a research and development process that can take as long as six to 12 years and can cost from $50 million to $300 million. The level of pre-market evaluation done on every biotechnology crop is far greater than for any other type of food crop. As previously mentioned, the monitoring and tests include both food safety and environmental impact assessments. In addition, the USDA, EPA and FDA each have the authority to recall products from the food chain if new science-based information identifies a public or environmental health hazard.

Second, I do not see this as an either/or situation, meaning organic verses biotech. Organic farming and conventional farming involving biotechnology can and do coexist. Biotechnology can make the food we eat safer, more nutritious and free from allergens. The use of biotechnology in agriculture has enhanced the well-being and environmental stewardship of communities through reduced pesticide use and exposure to other environmental factors. Allowing farmers the ability to choose what and how to grow is the very essence of free market. Organic and biotech choices are tools in a farmer's "toolbox" which allow for farmers to choose to utilize the widest range of technologies available to produce a safe, healthy, abundant and affordable food supply. In other words, there is no justification for restricting the farmers' ability to utilize the kind of breakthroughs and ingenuity we celebrate in every other facet of life. In a world of iPods, cell phones, Palm Pilots and GPS technology, why should farmers be made to use the outdated equivalents of cassette players, rotary phones, Rolodexes, and pre-satellite navigation?

No Evidence of Inferiority or Harm

Third, there is no evidence that organically produced food is any safer than food produced by any other method of farming, nor is there a clear nutritional bonus to eating organic. However, I uphold organic farming as an option for any farmer wishing to incorporate organic farming practices into their operations. In fact, I truly believe that organic products are enjoying great niche-market success, in part, because of misguided media hype that buys into propaganda that *The Future of Food* promulgates.

Fourth, there is no evidence that genetically engineered foods currently on the market pose any human health concern or that they are any less safe than those foods produced through traditional breeding. [The National Academy of Sciences reports,] "To date, no adverse health effects attributed to genetic engineering have been documented in the human population." Furthermore, no commercially available, genetically engineered food product contains genetic information of DNA sequence derived from an animal (i.e. fish-headed tomatoes are mythical).

Companies Must Use GM Foods

Six percent to 8 percent of children and 1 to 2 percent of adults are allergic to one or another food ingredient, and an estimated 150 Americans die each year from exposure to food allergens. Allergies to peanuts, soybeans, and wheat proteins, for example, are quite common and can be severe. Although only about 1 percent of the population is allergic to peanuts, some individuals are so highly sensitive that exposure causes anaphylactic shock, killing dozens of people every year in North America.

Protecting those with true food allergies is a daunting task. Farmers, food shippers and processors, wholesalers and retailers, and even restaurants must maintain meticulous records and labels and ensure against cross-contamination. Still, in a country where about a billion meals are eaten every day, missteps are inevitable. Dozens of processed food items must be recalled every year due to accidental contamination or inaccurate labeling.

Fortunately, biotechnology researchers are well along in the development of peanuts, soybeans, wheat, and other crops in which the genes coding for allergenic proteins have been silenced or removed. According to University of California, Berkeley, biochemist Bob Buchanan, hypoallergenic varieties of wheat could be ready for commercialization within the decade, and nuts soon thereafter. Once these products are commercially available, agricultural processors and food companies that refuse to use these safer food sources will open themselves to products-liability, design-defect lawsuits.

Henry I. Miller and Gregory Conko,
Policy Review, *June/July, 2006.*

A Reduction in Pesticide Use

Fifth, because of biotech crops, the world has benefited from a reduction in pesticide use. In the state-by-state study, *Impacts on U.S. Agriculture of Biotechnology-Derived Crops Planted in 2003*, conducted by the National Center for Food and Agriculture Policy, they evaluated biotechnology's impact on two of California's commodities—corn and cotton. The study concluded that the biotech varieties increased the state's food and fiber production by more than 10 million pounds, improved farm income by nearly $33 million and reduced pesticide use by 776,000 pounds annually. At a genetically modified foods debate at U.C. [University of California] Davis in October 2004, Professor Rick Rousch, Director of the Statewide Integrated Pest Management Program, cited studies that found pesticide poisonings among Chinese cotton workers have dropped by 75 percent, and insect resistant corn reduced the fungal toxins on insect-damaged corn in Africa where toxins are the likely culprit behind a high incidence of throat cancer and liver problems. Rousch also cited a 2001 European Union report that reviewed $65 million in research by some 400 research groups showing no new risks to human health or the environment compared to conventional plant breeding; and, in fact, that more precise technology and greater scrutiny probably made genetically modified (GM) crops safer than conventional ones. Plant biotechnology provides new options for Integrated Pest Management (IPM) programs, reduces the overall use of pesticides and enables soil-conserving management practices.

Sadly, the ideology behind many organic supporters is not backed by sound science, or even a love for the land. Many biotech foes oppose the industrialization of the agricultural industry, yet few have actually farmed or have a true understanding of agriculture other than a trip to the grocery store. An all orgranic world is neither "sustainable" nor an efficient use of the land. Organic farming is less efficient and certified organic produce is more expensive than traditionally farmed produce. By comparison, traditional or conventional farmers incorporate many technologies into their cultural practices to achieve sustainable agricultural that is often rejected by many organic farmers. . . .

Other Myths

Cross-Contamination: Regarding pollen drift/gene-flow, organic growers will not lose their certification if their crop shows GM variety within their crop. If the grower demonstrates that his/her organic plan has the appropriate safeguards in place to attempt to avoid contamination, the grower's certification cannot be revoked. If the certifier denies the grower's organic status, the grower can appeal the decision, and the California Department of Food and Agriculture will grant it back, so long as the grower maintains his/her normal organic-growing practices.

Several California farmers successfully farm conventional, organic and biotech crops. They do so by creating buffers between crop varietals and implementing practices such as crop rotation and monitoring.

Royalties: The film criticizes royalties paid to seed companies for the use of their seed. In the agricultural industry, royalties are paid for conventional, organic and biotech varieties of commodities such as peaches, plums, cotton and roses. For example, a farmer may pay a royalty fee to the University of California for a stone fruit variety they developed; the royalty fee helps to offset their research costs and funds further research.

Seed Harvesting: Seventy-five percent of the world's farmers save seed, but in the United States it is only about ten percent. In other parts of the world, they are saving seed because they do not have access or resources to the commercial varieties. . . .

Superweed: In regard to the creation of a superweed [plant created when a weed crosses with a GM crop and becomes resistant to herbicides] good cultural practices dictate the rotation of crops and implements to prevent resistance or tiring of the soil. If all scientific advances were halted out of fear of the unknown, life-saving technological breakthroughs such as penicillin, the pasteurization of milk, or the polio vaccine would have never been made available to the world.

World Acceptance: World cultivation of plants from modern biotechnology is increasing year by year. More than seven million farmers in eighteen countries planted a total of 167.2 million acres in 2003, up fifteen percent from 2002. At present, there are about sixteen varieties approved for commercial cultivation. The four major countries are Argentina, Canada, China and the United States.

Exaggerated Fear Campaign: *The Future of Food* is just another exploit in a long line of many acts of hype. North Dakota wheat farmer Al Skogen fervently describes his opinion of the environmental movement against biotech, "It's clear to most farmers that the environmental movement completely has neglected the fact that biotech crops are a solid step forward for the environment. Unfortunately, most environmental activist groups sold their allegiance to the environment a long time ago in exchange for a fully funded fear campaign supported by trust funders, organic promoters and professional agitators."

Consumers Deserve a Choice

I believe farmers should retain as much choice as possible in determining what they plant, and consumers should have an equal amount of freedom in choosing what they eat.

As a farmer, I look to biotechnology in hopes that research will avail new types of crops and livestock that improve product quality, reduce labor, reduce insecticide use, reduce soil erosion, improve air and water quality, etc. In addition to increased yields and less environmental impacts, I can anticipate better health because I will no longer be exposed to certain insecticides when growing insect-resistant biotech crops.

As a consumer and a mother, I believe biotech or genetically modified foods can offer lower prices, better nutrition and fewer pesticide residues. So, I will continue to buy them without hesitation. In the same manner, I will also continue to exercise my freedom of choice to purchase organically and conventionally grown foods and products as I see fit.

Biotechnology is not the silver bullet and it is not without its shortcomings. However, with an increasing world population and rampant disease in third-world countries, I am confident research will continue to "grow" solutions that will benefit us all. It is a powerful tool to increase food production, protect the environment, improve the nutritional value of food, and produce invaluable pharmaceuticals. I encourage you to educate yourself on the issue and make your own informed decision on the biotech issue. I am confident you will reach a similar, if not the same, conclusion I did.

"Scientists have identified a number of ways in which genetically engineered organisms could potentially adversely impact both human health and the environment."

The Safeness of Genetically Modified Foods Is Unproven

Union of Concerned Scientists

In the following viewpoint, the Union of Concerned Scientists (UCS) argues that the health and environmental risks associated with the use of genetically modified (GM) crops is substantial. The organization maintains that at the present time, the knowledge base scientists need to fully assess the impact of GM crops is incomplete. Therefore, no one is sure what harmful effects GM crops might have on consumers or the environment. The Union of Concerned Scientists is a science-based, nonprofit environmental organization.

As you read, consider the following questions:

1. According to the Union for Concerned Scientists, what are two ways in which genetically engineered plants could result in human resistance to antibiotics?

Union of Concerned Scientists, "Risks of Genetic Engineering," June 6, 2007. www.ucs usa.org. Reproduced by permission.

2. In the author's view, what types of toxic materials may increase in plants as a result of genetic engineering?

3. What are some of the potential negative reactions the UCS suggests could occur as a result of interaction between genetically modified plants and native plants?

Many previous technologies have proved to have adverse effects unexpected by their developers. DDT [a synthetic pesticide now banned for agricultural use worldwide], for example, turned out to accumulate in fish and thin the shells of fish-eating birds like eagles and ospreys. And chlorofluorocarbons [chemical compounds previously used in refrigerants, propellants, and cleaning solvents, but now used only if no alternative exists] turned out to float into the upper atmosphere and destroy ozone, a chemical that shields the earth from dangerous radiation. What harmful effects might turn out to be associated with the use or release of genetically engineered organisms?

This is not an easy question. Being able to answer it depends on understanding complex biological and ecological systems. So far, scientists know of no generic harms associated with genetically engineered organisms. For example, it is *not* true that *all* genetically engineered foods are toxic or that *all* released engineered organisms are likely to proliferate in the environment. But specific engineered organisms may be harmful by virtue of the novel gene combinations they possess. This means that the risks of genetically engineered organisms must be assessed case by case and that these risks can differ greatly from one gene-organism combination to another.

So far, scientists have identified a number of ways in which genetically engineered organisms could potentially adversely impact both human health and the environment. Once the potential harms are identified, the question becomes how likely are they to occur. The answer to this question falls into the arena of risk assessment.

In addition to posing risks of harm that we can envision and attempt to assess, genetic engineering may also pose risks that we simply do not know enough to identify. The recognition of this possibility does not by itself justify stopping the technology, but does put a substantial burden on those who wish to go forward to demonstrate benefits.

Here are some examples of the potential adverse effects [that] genetically engineered organisms may have on human health. Most of these examples are associated with the growth and consumption of genetically engineered crops. Different risks would be associated with genetically engineered animals and, like the risks associated with plants, would depend largely on the new traits introduced into the organism.

Safe Food Becomes Allergenic

Transgenic crops could bring new allergens into foods that sensitive individuals would not know to avoid. An example is transferring the gene for one of the many allergenic proteins found in milk into vegetables like carrots. Mothers who know to avoid giving their sensitive children milk would not know to avoid giving them transgenic carrots containing milk proteins. The problem is unique to genetic engineering because it alone can transfer proteins across species boundaries into completely unrelated organisms.

Genetic engineering routinely moves proteins into the food supply from organisms that have never been consumed as foods. Some of those proteins could be food allergens, since virtually all known food allergens are proteins. Recent research substantiates concerns about genetic engineering rendering previously safe foods allergenic. A study by scientists at the University of Nebraska shows that soybeans genetically engineered to contain Brazil-nut proteins cause reactions in individuals allergic to Brazil nuts.

Scientists have limited ability to predict whether a particular protein will be a food allergen, if consumed by humans.

The only sure way to determine whether protein will be an allergen is through experience. Thus importing proteins, particularly from nonfood sources, is a gamble with respect to their allergenicity.

Potential for Resistance to Antibiotics

Genetic engineering often uses genes for antibiotic resistance as "selectable markers." Early in the engineering process, these markers help select cells that have taken up foreign genes. Although they have no further use, the genes continue to be expressed in plant tissues. Most genetically engineered plant foods carry fully functioning antibiotic-resistance genes.

The presence of antibiotic-resistance genes in foods could have two harmful effects. First, eating these foods could reduce the effectiveness of antibiotics to fight disease when these antibiotics are taken with meals. Antibiotic-resistance genes produce enzymes that can degrade antibiotics. If a tomato with an antibiotic-resistance gene is eaten at the same time as an antibiotic, it could destroy the antibiotic in the stomach.

Second, the resistance genes could be transferred to human or animal pathogens, making them impervious to antibiotics. If transfer were to occur, it could aggravate the already serious health problem of antibiotic-resistant disease organisms. Although unmediated transfers of genetic material from plants to bacteria are highly unlikely, any possibility that they may occur requires careful scrutiny in light of the seriousness of antibiotic resistance.

In addition, the widespread presence of antibiotic-resistance genes in engineered food suggests that as the number of genetically engineered products grows, the effects of antibiotic resistance should be analyzed cumulatively across the food supply.

Increasing Toxic Materials in Plants

Many organisms have the ability to produce toxic substances. For plants, such substances help to defend stationary organisms from the many predators in their environment. In some cases, plants contain inactive pathways leading to toxic substances. Addition of new genetic material through genetic engineering could reactivate these inactive pathways or otherwise increase the levels of toxic substances within the plants. This could happen, for example, if the on/off signals associated with the introduced gene were located on the genome in places where they could turn on the previously inactive genes.

Some of the new genes being added to crops can remove heavy metals like mercury from the soil and concentrate them in the plant tissue. The purpose of creating such crops is to make possible the use of municipal sludge as fertilizer. Sludge contains useful plant nutrients, but often cannot be used as fertilizer because it is contaminated with toxic heavy metals. The idea is to engineer plants to remove and sequester those metals in inedible parts of plants. In a tomato, for example, the metals would be sequestered in the roots; in potatoes in the leaves. Turning on the genes in only some parts of the plants requires the use of genetic on/off switches that turn on only in specific tissues, like leaves.

Such products pose risks of contaminating foods with high levels of toxic metals if the on/off switches are not completely turned off in edible tissues. There are also environmental risks associated with the handling and disposal of the metal-contaminated parts of plants after harvesting.

Although for the most part health risks are the result of the genetic material newly added to organisms, it is also possible for the removal of genes and gene products to cause problems. For example, genetic engineering might be used to produce decaffeinated coffee beans by deleting or turning off genes associated with caffeine production. But caffeine helps protect coffee beans against fungi. Beans that are unable to

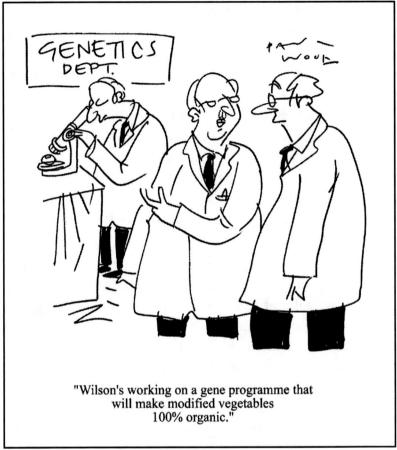

"Wilson's working on a gene programme that will make modified vegetable 100% organic," cartoon by Paul Wood, CartoonStock.com

produce caffeine might be coated with fungi, which can produce toxins. Fungal toxins, such as aflatoxin, are potent human toxins that can remain active through processes of food preparation.

As with any new technology, the full set of risks associated with genetic engineering have almost certainly not been identified. The ability to imagine what might go wrong with a technology is limited by the currently incomplete understanding of physiology, genetics, and nutrition.

Invasion of the Natural Environment

One way of thinking generally about the environmental harm that genetically engineered plants might do is to consider that they might become weeds. Here, weeds means all plants in places where humans do not want them. The term covers everything from Johnson grass choking crops in fields to kudzu blanketing trees to melaleuca trees invading the Everglades. In each case, the plants are growing unaided by humans in places where they are having unwanted effects. In agriculture, weeds can severely inhibit crop yield. In unmanaged environments, like the Everglades, invading trees can displace natural flora and upset whole ecosystems.

Some weeds result from the accidental introduction of alien plants, but many were the result of purposeful introductions for agricultural and horticultural purposes. Some of the plants intentionally introduced into the United States that have become serious weeds are Johnson grass, multiflora rose, and kudzu. A new combination of traits produced as a result of genetic engineering might enable crops to thrive unaided in the environment in circumstances where they would then be considered new or worse weeds. One example would be a rice plant engineered to be salt-tolerant that escaped cultivation and invaded nearby marine estuaries.

Novel genes placed in crops will not necessarily stay in agricultural fields. If relatives of the altered crops are growing near the field, the new gene can easily move via pollen into those plants. The new traits might confer on wild or weedy relatives of crop plants the ability to thrive in unwanted places, making them weeds as defined above. For example, a gene changing the oil composition of a crop might move into nearby weedy relatives in which the new oil composition would enable the seeds to survive the winter. Overwintering might allow the plant to become a weed or might intensify weedy properties it already possesses.

Rendering Pesticides Useless

Crops genetically engineered to be resistant to chemical herbicides are tightly linked to the use of particular chemical pesticides. Adoption of these crops could therefore lead to changes in the mix of chemical herbicides used across the country. To the extent that chemical herbicides differ in their environmental toxicity, these changing patterns could result in greater levels of environmental harm overall. In addition, widespread use of herbicide-tolerant crops could lead to the rapid evolution of resistance to herbicides in weeds, either as a result of increased exposure to the herbicide or as a result of the transfer of the herbicide trait to weedy relatives of crops. Again, since herbicides differ in their environmental harm, loss of some herbicides may be detrimental to the environment overall.

Many insects contain genes that render them susceptible to pesticides. Often these susceptibility genes predominate in natural populations of insects. These genes are a valuable natural resource because they allow pesticides to remain as effective pest-control tools. The more benign the pesticide, the more valuable the genes that make pests susceptible to it.

Certain genetically engineered crops threaten the continued susceptibility of pests to one of nature's most valuable pesticides: the *Bacillus thuringiensis* or Bt toxin. These "Bt crops" are genetically engineered to contain a gene for the Bt toxin. Because the crops produce the toxin in most plant tissues throughout the life cycle of the plant, pests are constantly exposed to it. This continuous exposure selects for the rare resistance genes in the pest population and in time will render the Bt pesticide useless, unless specific measures are instituted to avoid the development of such resistance.

Harming Other Plants and Animals

Addition of foreign genes to plants could also have serious consequences for wildlife in a number of circumstances. For example, engineering crop plants, such as tobacco or rice, to produce plastics or pharmaceuticals could endanger mice or deer who consume crop debris left in the fields after harvesting. Fish that have been engineered to contain metal-sequestering proteins (such fish have been suggested as living pollution clean-up devices) could be harmful if consumed by other fish or raccoons.

One of the most common applications of genetic engineering is the production of virus-tolerant crops. Such crops are produced by engineering components of viruses into the plant genomes. For reasons not well understood, plants producing viral components on their own are resistant to subsequent infection by those viruses. Such plants, however, pose other risks of creating new or worse viruses through two mechanisms: recombination and transcapsidation.

Recombination can occur between the plant-produced viral genes and closely related genes of incoming viruses. Such recombination may produce viruses that can infect a wider range of hosts or that may be more virulent than the parent viruses.

Transcapsidation involves the encapsulation of the genetic material of one virus by the plant-produced viral proteins. Such hybrid viruses could transfer viral genetic material to a new host plant that it could not otherwise infect. Except in rare circumstances, this would be a one-time-only effect, because the viral genetic material carries no genes for the foreign proteins within which it was encapsulated and would not be able to produce a second generation of hybrid viruses.

As with human health risks, it is unlikely that all potential harms to the environment have been identified. Each of the potential harms above is an answer to the question, "Well, what might go wrong?" The answer to that question depends on how well scientists understand the organism and the environment into which it is released. At this point, biology and ecology are too poorly understood to be certain that question has been answered comprehensively.

> "Bioengineering . . . can be used to ad-
> vance food security while promoting
> sustainable agriculture."

Genetically Modified Crops Can Help End World Hunger

Gregory Conko and C.S. Prakash

In the following viewpoint, Gregory Conko and C.S. Prakash argue that genetically modified (GM) crops offer a promising solution to the global problem of hunger. The authors outline the benefits of GM crops and contrast GM farming with traditional plant breeding methods and organic farming. They assert that criticism of GM farming results from a lack of knowledge or a fear of the unknown. Gregory Conko is the director of the public interest group Competitive Enterprise Institute as well as vice president of the AgBioWorld Foundation. C.S. Prakash is founder and president of the AgBioWorld Foundation and a professor of plant biotechnology at Tuskegee University in Alabama.

As you read, consider the following questions:

1. According to Conko and Prakash, how many people go to bed on an empty stomach, and how many people die every day as a result of hunger or related problems?

Gregory Conko and C.S. Prakash, "Can GM Crops Play a Role in Developing Countries?" *PBI Bulletin*, no. 2, 2004. Reproduced by permission.

2. Why, according to the authors, is organic farming inferior to GM farming?

3. What are the potential benefits of GM crops as outlined by Conko and Prakash?

In 2002, while more than 14 million people in six drought-stricken southern African countries faced the risk of starvation, efforts by the U.N.'s World Food Programme were stifled by the global "GM" [genetically modified] food controversy. Food aid, containing kernels of bioengineered corn from the United States, was initially rejected by all six governments, even though the very same corn has been consumed daily by hundreds of millions in North and South America and has been distributed by the World Food Programme throughout Africa since 1996.

Four of those governments later accepted the grain on condition that it be milled to prevent planting, but Zimbabwe and Zambia continue to refuse it to this day [2004], and recently Angola also joined this group. Zambian President Levy Mwanawasa said [in 2002 that] his people would rather starve than eat bioengineered food, which he described as "poison." The actually starving Zambian people felt differently, though. One news report after another described scenes of hungry Zambians rioting and overpowering armed guards trying to release tens of thousands of tons of the corn locked away in warehouses by the government.

This is one of the tragic consequences of global fearmongering about recombinant DNA technology and bioengineered crops. Although many varieties that are of use to resource-poor farmers in less developed countries are at very early stages of the development process, even ones that have already been commercialized in such countries as Canada and the United States are being kept from farmers by governments skeptical of "genetic modification".

Risks Not Limited to GM Crops

In the most fundamental sense, however, all plant and animal breeding involves—and always has involved—the intentional genetic modification of organisms. And though critics of recombinant DNA believe it is unique, there have always been Cassandras [term taken from Greek mythology that refers to a person who is always predicting that something bad is to come] to claim that the latest technology was unnatural, different from its predecessors, and inherently dangerous.

As early as 1906, Luther Burbank, the noted plant breeder, said that "we have recently advanced our knowledge of genetics to the point where we can manipulate life in a way never intended by nature, We must proceed with the utmost caution in the application of this new found knowledge," a quip that one might just as easily hear today regarding recombinant DNA modification.

But just as Burbank was wrong to claim that there was some special danger in knowledge or technology, so are today's skeptics wrong to believe that modern genetic modification poses some inherent risk. It is not genetic modification per se that generates risk. Recombinant DNA–modified, conventionally modified, and unmodified plants could all prove to be invasive, harm biodiversity, or be harmful to eat. It is not the technique used to modify organisms that makes them risky. Rather risk arises from the characteristics of individual organisms, as well as how and where they are used.

That is why the use of bioengineering technology for the development of improved plant varieties has been endorsed by dozens of scientific bodies. The UN's Food and Agriculture Organization (FAO) and World Health Organization, the UK's [United Kingdom's] Royal Society, the American Medical Association, and the French Academies of Medicine and Science, among others, have studied bioengineering techniques and given them a clean bill of health. Moreover, bioengineered crop plants may be of even greater value in less developed countries than in industrialized ones.

A Weapon in the Fight to End Hunger

In a report published in July 2000, the UK's Royal Society, the National Academies of Science from Brazil, China, India, Mexico, and the U.S., and the Third World Academy of Science, embraced bioengineering, arguing that it can be used to advance food security while promoting sustainable agriculture. "It is critical," declared the scientists, "that the potential benefits of GM technology become available to developing countries." And an FAO report issued in May 2004 argued that "effective transfer of existing technologies to poor rural communities and the development of new and safe biotechnologies can greatly enhance the prospects for sustainably improving agricultural productivity today and in the future," as well as "help reduce environmental damage caused by toxic agricultural chemicals."

Today, some 740 million people go to bed daily on an empty stomach, and nearly 40,000 people—half of them children—die every day due to hunger or malnutrition-related causes. Despite commitments by industrialized countries to increase international aid, Africa still is expected to have over 180 million undernourished citizens in 2030, according to a report published [in 2004] by the UN Millennium Project Task Force. Although bioengineered crops alone will not eliminate hunger, they can provide a useful tool for addressing the many agricultural problems in Africa, Asia, Latin America, and other poor tropical regions.

Indeed, recombinant DNA-modified crops have already increased crop yields and food production, and reduced the use of synthetic chemical pesticides in both industrialized and less developed countries. These advances are critical in a world where natural resources are finite and where hundreds of millions of people suffer from hunger and malnutrition. Critics dismiss such claims as nothing more than corporate public relations puffery. However, while it is true that most commercially available bioengineered plants were designed for farmers in the industrialized world, the increasing adoption of biotech varieties by underdeveloped countries over the past few years demonstrates their broader applicability.

Globally, bioengineered varieties are now grown on more than 165 million acres (67.7 million hectares) in 18 countries, such as Argentina, Australia, Brazil, Canada, China, India, Mexico, the Philippines, South Africa, and the United States, according to the International Service for the Acquisition of Agri-Biotech Applications (ISAAA). Nearly one-quarter of that acreage is farmed by some 6 million resource-poor farmers in less developed countries. Why? Because they see many of the same benefits that farmers in industrialized nations do.

Resistance to Pests and Disease

The first generation of biotech crops—approximately 50 different varieties of canola, corn, cotton, potato, squash, soybean, and others—were designed to aid in protecting crops from insect pests, weeds, and plant diseases. As much as 40 percent of crop productivity in Africa and Asia and about 20 percent in the industrialized countries of North America and Europe is lost to these biotic stresses, despite the use of large amounts of insecticides, herbicides, and other agricultural chemicals. Poor tropical farmers may face different pest species than their industrial country counterparts, but both must constantly battle against these threats to their productivity.

That's why South African and Filipino farmers are so eager to grow bioengineered corn resistant to insect pests, and why Chinese, Indian, and South African farmers like biotech insect-resistant cotton so much. Indian cotton farmers and Brazilian and Paraguayan soy growers didn't even wait for their governments to approve biotech varieties before they began growing them. It was discovered in 2001 that Indian farmers were planting seed obtained illegally from field trials of a biotech cotton variety then still under governmental review. Farmers in Brazil and Paraguay looked across the border and saw how well their Argentine neighbors were doing with transgenic soybean varieties and smuggling of bioengineered seed became rampant.

When the Indian government finally approved bioengineered cotton in 2002 for cultivation in seven southern states it proved to be highly successful. A study conducted by the University of Agriculture in Dharwad [India] found that more insect damage was done to conventional hybrids than to the bioengineered variety and that the bioengineered cotton reduced pesticide spraying by half or more, delivering a 30–40 percent profit increase.

During the 2002–2003 growing season, some Indian cotton farmers saw no increased yield from the more expensive biotech varieties, but droughts during that year generated harsh conditions throughout India's southern cotton belt. Many growers of conventional crop varieties also suffered unanticipated and tragic crop losses. Most of the farmers who grew bioengineered cotton decided to plant it again in 2003, however, and total planted acreage grew from approximately 1 million acres in 2002–2003 to an estimated 3.3 million acres in 2003–2004.

Benefits of GM Crops

When the planting of bioengineered soybean was provisionally legalized in Brazil for the 2003–2004 growing season, over 50,000 farmers registered their intent to plant it—including almost 98 percent of the growers in the southern-most state of Rio Grande do Sul, where the soybeans originally bred for Argentine climatic conditions will grow best. What is especially noteworthy is that the government decree did not legalize commercial sales of the biotech soybean, it only authorized the planting of illegal seed already in the possession of farm-

Americans' Approval of Genetically Modified (GM) Foods Based on Knowledge of GM Foods

In a phone survey of 1,200 noninstitutionalized adults, participants were asked 12 questions to assess their knowledge of genetically modified foods. Answering 1-5 questions correctly led to a classification of "low score," answering 6-9 questions correctly resulted in a classification of "medium score," and answering 10-12 questions correctly placed a respondent in the "high score" category.

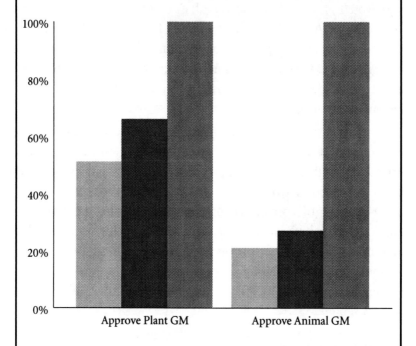

Low Score
Medium Score
High Score

TAKEN FROM: Venkata Puduri, Ramu Govindasamy, John T. Lang, and Benjamin Ohyango, "I Will Not Eat It with a Fox; I Will Not Eat It in a Box: What Determines Acceptance of GM Food for American Consumers?" *Choices*, 4th Quarter 2005.

ers. Thus, by registering their intent to grow the bioengineered variety, farmers were informing the government of their prior guilt.

There are few greater testaments to the benefits of biotechnology than the fact that thousands of poor farmers are willing to acknowledge having committed a crime just to gain access to the improved varieties. The clear lesson is that, where bioengineered varieties become available (legal or not), most farmers themselves are eager to try them.

There is even evidence that biotech varieties have literally saved human lives. In less developed nations, pesticides are typically sprayed on crops by hand, exposing farm workers to severe health risks. Some 400 to 500 Chinese cotton farmers die every year from acute pesticide poisoning because, until recently, the only alternative was risking near total crop loss due to voracious insects. A study conducted by researchers at the Chinese Academy of Sciences and Rutgers University in the U.S. found that adoption of bioengineered cotton varieties in China has lowered the amount of pesticides used by more than 75 percent and reduced the number of pesticide poisonings by an equivalent amount. Another study by economists at the University of Reading in the UK found that South African cotton farmers have seen similar benefits.

The productivity gains generated by bioengineered crops provide yet another important benefit: they could save millions of acres of sensitive wildlife habitat from being converted into farmland. The loss and fragmentation of wildlife habitats caused by agricultural encroachment in regions experiencing the greatest population growth are widely recognized as among the most serious threats to biodiversity. Thus, increasing agricultural productivity is an essential environmental goal, and one that would be much easier in a world where bioengineering technology is in widespread use.

Organic Farming Cannot Compete

Opponents of biotechnology argue that organic farming can reduce pesticide use even more than bioengineered crops can. But organic farming practices are less productive, because there are few effective organic controls for insects, weeds, or pathogens. Converting from modern, technology-based agriculture to organic would mean either reducing global food output significantly or sacrificing undeveloped land to agriculture. Moreover, feeding the anticipated population of eight or nine billion people in the year 2050 will mean increasing food production by at least 50 percent.

As it is, the annual rate of increase in food production globally has dropped from 3 percent in the 1970s to 1 percent today. Additional gains from conventional breeding are certainly possible, but the maximum theoretical yields for most crop plants are being approached rapidly. Despite the simplistic claims made by critics of plant technology, providing genuine food security must include solutions other than mere redistribution. There is simply no way for organic farming to feed a global population of nine billion people without having to bring substantially more land into agricultural use. Dramatically improving crop yields will prove to be an essential environmental and humanitarian goal.

We have already realized significant environmental benefits from the biotech crops currently being grown, including a reduction in pesticide use of 20 million kg [kilograms] in the U.S. alone. A 2002 Council for Agricultural Science and Technology report also found that recombinant DNA–modified crops in the U.S. promote the adoption of conservation tillage practices, resulting in many other important environmental benefits: 37 million tons of topsoil preserved; 85 percent reduction in greenhouse gas emissions from farm machinery; 70 percent reduction in herbicide run-off, 90 percent decrease in soil erosion; and from 15 to 26 liters of fuel saved per acre.

And, as we have seen, while the first generation of bioengineered crops was not designed with poor tropical farmers in mind, these varieties are highly adaptable. Examples of the varieties that now are being designed specifically for resource-poor farmers include virus-resistant cassava, insect-resistant rice, sweet potato, and pigeon pea, and dozens of others. Chinese scientists, leaders in the development of both bioengineered and conventional rice have been urging their governments to approve commercialization of their biotech varieties that have been thoroughly tested and ready for market for several years.

The Unlimited Potential of GM Crops

The next generation of products, now in research labs and field trial plots, includes crops designed to tolerate climatic stresses such as extremes of heat, cold, and drought, as well as crops designed to grow better in poor tropical soils high in acidity or alkalinity, or contaminated with mineral salts. A Mexican research group has shown that tropical crops can be modified using recombinant DNA technology to better tolerate acidic soils, significantly increasing the productivity of corn, rice and papaya. These traits for greater tolerance to adverse environmental conditions would be tremendously advantageous to poor farmers in less developed countries, especially those in Africa.

Africa did not benefit from the Green Revolution as much as Asian and Latin American nations did because plant breeders focused on improving crops such as rice and wheat, which are not widely grown in Africa. Plus, much of the African dry lands have little rainfall and no potential for irrigation, both of which play essential roles in productivity success stories for crops such as Asian rice. And the remoteness of many African villages and the poor transportation infrastructure in land-locked African countries make it difficult for African farmers to obtain agricultural chemical inputs such as fertilizers, insecticides and herbicides—even if they could be donated by aid agencies and charities. But, by packaging technological inputs within seeds, biotechnology can provide the same, or better, productivity advantages as chemical or mechanical inputs, but in a much more user-friendly manner. Farmers could be able to control insect pests, viral or bacterial pathogens, extremes of heat or drought and poor soil quality, just by planting these crops.

And the now-famous Golden Rice, with added beta carotene, is just one of many examples of bioengineered crops with improved nutritional content. Indian scientists have recently announced development of a new high-protein potato variety available for commercial cultivation. Another team of Indian scientists, working with technical and financial assistance from Monsanto, is developing an improved mustard variety with enhanced beta-carotene in its oil. One lab at Tuskegee University is enhancing the level of dietary protein in sweet potatoes, a common staple crop in sub-Saharan Africa. Researchers are also developing varieties of cassava, rice, and corn that more efficiently absorb trace metals and micronutrients from the soil, have enhanced starch quality, and contain more beta-carotene and other beneficial vitamins and minerals.

Only Fear Is Standing in the Way

Ultimately, while no assurance of perfect safety can be made, breeders know far more about the genetic makeup, product characteristics, and safety of every modern bioengineered crop than those of any conventional variety ever marketed. Breeders know exactly what new genetic material has been introduced. They can identify where the transferred genes have been inserted into the new plant. They can test to ensure that transferred genes are working properly and that the nutritional elements of the food have been unchanged. None of these safety assurances have ever before been made with conventional breeding techniques. We have always lived with food risks. But modern genetic technology makes it increasingly easier to reduce those risks.

Societal anxiety over the new tools for genetic modification is, in some ways, understandable. It is fueled by a variety of causes, including consumer unfamiliarity, lack of reliable information on the current safeguards in place, a steady stream of negative opinion in the news media, opposition by activist groups, growing mistrust of industry, and a general lack of awareness of how our food production system has evolved over time. But saying that public apprehension over biotechnology is understandable is not the same as saying that it is valid. With more than thirty years of experience using recombinant DNA technology, and nearly two decades worth of pre-commercial and commercial experience with bioengineered crop plants, we can be confident that it is one of the most important and safe technologies in the plant breeder's toolbox. It would be a shame to deny biotechnology's fruits to those who are most in need of its benefits.

"The problem of hunger in developing countries is not caused by lack of genetic engineering to produce more food."

Genetically Modified Crops Will Not End World Hunger

Carl F. Jordan

In the following viewpoint, Carl F. Jordan argues that genetically modified (GM) crops will not sufficiently address the causes and problems associated with world hunger. He contends that economic, government, and social problems are at the root of hunger, not just a lack of food. Additionally, Jordan states that continued focus on GM crops has led policy makers to ignore alternative solutions that may provide greater benefit to those in need. Carl F. Jordan is a senior research scientist and professor at the University of Georgia.

As you read, consider the following questions:

1. What does the author identify as the causes of hunger?

2. According to Jordan, how will the introduction of transgenic crops impact indigenous cultures and crops?

Carl F. Jordan, "Genetic Engineering, the Farm Crisis, and World Hunger," *BioScience*, vol. 52, no. 6, June 2002, pp. 523–29. Republished with permission of BioScience, conveyed through Copyright Clearance Center, Inc.

3. What are some of the alternative approaches to combating hunger suggested by the author?

There has always been hunger somewhere in the world, but the belief that it is a problem that developed countries should solve is relatively recent. Only after World War II, when pesticides, herbicides, and inorganic fertilizers became readily available, was it even possible to think that world hunger could be alleviated. To do the job, however, it was necessary to breed crops that could take advantage of these new chemicals. The term Green Revolution has been used to signify the introduction of these crops, along with the necessary infrastructure (tractors, cultivation equipment, irrigation systems) in underdeveloped countries.

There are claims of impressive gains in food production as a result of the Green Revolution, especially in Southeast Asia. During two decades of Green Revolution advances (1970-1990), figures from the United Nations show that the total food available per person in the world rose by 11 percent, while the estimated number of hungry people fell from 942 million to 786 million, a 16 percent drop. This was apparent progress, for which those behind the Green Revolution took credit. But if China (where Green Revolution techniques were not emphasized and employed) is eliminated from the analysis, the number of hungry people in the rest of the world actually increased by more than 11 percent, from 536 million to 597 million. In South America, for example, while per capita food supplies rose almost 8 percent, the number of hungry people also went up by 19 percent.

World population continues to grow, while food production resulting from the first Green Revolution is tapering off and may have reached its ceiling. As a result, there has been a call for a second Green Revolution. Genetically altered plants have been proclaimed to be the key to this revolution that will stave off future world shortages of food. In an article in *Science*, Ismail Serageldin, vice president for special programs at the World Bank, made a strong pitch for further development of genetically modified crops. He quoted figures that showed average grain yields throughout the world must increase by 80 percent over the 1990 average to meet projected food demands by 2025. An important strategy, he says, is harnessing the genetic revolution, with cutting-edge work associated with gene mapping, molecular markers, and biotechnology. . . .

The Causes of Hunger

The problem of hunger in developing countries is not caused by lack of genetic engineering to produce more food. In most countries where hunger is prevalent, there is an excess of staples—"the world already produces sufficient food" [states expert Nikos Alexandratos]. Today, there is enough grain produced to provide every human being on the planet with thirty-five hundred calories a day. This estimate does not even count many other commonly eaten foods such as vegetables, beans, nuts, root crops, fruits, meat from grass-fed animals, and fish.

[Argues Alexandratos,] "The undernourished and the food-insecure [lacking a stable food supply] persons are in these conditions because they are poor in terms of income to purchase food, or in terms of access to agricultural resources, education, technology, infrastructure, and credit to produce their own food." Even in rich countries there are urban and rural ghettos where poverty, not lack of food, is the problem.

During the last two decades on through the beginning of the 21st century, there have been many countries whose people have suffered deprivation and starvation caused by political upheavals. Sudan [in Africa] is an example. According to the *New York Times*, an estimated two million Sudanese have died during 17 years of famine, caused by a war between the Arabs in the north and the people in the south of the country over the southern oil deposits. In the 1990s, tens of thousands of hungry Afghans moved to Herat, near the border of Iran, driven by civil war, bad government, and drought. In 2001, they fled to Pakistan. In the Congo, people are fleeing into Zambia, where Angolans also seek shelter. The small nation of Guinea is being overwhelmed by hundreds of thousands of people fleeing a cruel government in Liberia and a civil war in Sierra Leone.

[Agricultural ecologist Gordon] Conway has summarized other reasons that, despite the Green Revolution, hunger continues in developing countries: economic policies that discriminate against agriculture; restricted markets for farm inputs and outputs; inefficient rural financial institutions, including inadequate access by farmers to credit, inputs, and marketing services; lack of land reform or redistribution; inadequate rural infrastructure, including irrigation, transport, and marketing; lack of investment in rural education, clean water, health, nutrition programs, and family planning; lack of attention to the needs and legal rights of women and ethnic minorities; and lack of development and dissemination of appropriate agricultural technologies.

If these problems are ignored, there is no possibility that world hunger can be alleviated. If these problems were to be solved, then indeed increased production could be helpful. But it is not clear that genetically engineered crops are necessary to achieve this increase. In the report "Agriculture: Towards 2015/30, Technical Interim Report, April 2000," researchers in the Economic and Social Department at the Food and Agriculture Organization of the United Nations concluded that the world can produce enough food to meet global demands using current agricultural techniques. Their conclusion does not allow for any production improvements from genetically modified crops.

"Secret Knowledge" in the Sahel

What happens when technological development programs are instituted without attention to social, cultural, and economic aspects? A case study of traditional rice producers in the Sahel of Africa provides an illustration.

The climate in the Sahel region of Africa, made up in part by what is now Mali and Niger, is very dry. Average rainfall is less than 600 mm [millimeters] per year. As a result, the welfare of the Marka, a local ethnic group who are experts in the cultivation of rice, is highly influenced by climatic fluctuations. They have been cultivating native rice since prehistoric times, and they make complex and sophisticated decisions about when to plant and what varieties to plant. Their decisions are influenced by environmental clues—different varieties of rice have different vegetative periods, different adaptations to various flood depths, flood timing, pH tolerance, and fish predation. Different varieties are sown at different time intervals on different soil types.

The knowledge that the Marka possess about rice and its cultivation is secret and has been developed over a long period of time. It is a means of maintaining a specific ethnic identity. Social relations with other groups have become instituted as buffering mechanisms against potential bad times, allowing trade to occur without the necessity of immediate equal compensation. This buffering is useful, for example, with the Bozo fishers, who trade labor, goods, and services with the Marka. The buffering is beneficial to both groups, because weather that favors one group may disfavor the other.

Another important aspect of the Marka system is prioritized tenure on property held in common with the entire ethnic group. A hierarchical system prioritizes access to land, and the rules regulating access to common property have been encoded into local Islamic law. Prioritized access ensures that those with the specialized knowledge are those that make decisions on varieties of rice to be planted, as well as the timing of the planting.

Ensuring sustainability of rice production requires a deep understanding of how various social systems work. Social systems have deep ties to the environment through culturally mediated and specialized relationships. To know the physical needs of a particular crop is not enough information to produce consistent quantities in a sustainable manner. Farmers make decisions based on variables that may seem "unscientific," because the farmers are considering these variables from a different temporal and spatial scale than normally understood in the developed world. One needs to understand the evolutionary nature of "secret knowledge" and intergroup relations that function together as part of a subsistence system and that buffer the system against environmental and political variability.

The Degradation of Local Culture

Regional development projects in the Sahel break down this system of rice production. The goals of regional development projects are to increase the national market economy through production of rice and to technically mediate the uncertainty of the climate so as to guarantee a more steady supply to the market. Development programs usually require a change in cultivars from indigenous rice varieties to the Asian variety of rice, *Oryza sativa*, which is more marketable and has a higher yield, but requires consistent amounts of water. The knowledge about Asian rice is held by outsiders and is not secret. As a result of development, prioritized tenure on commonly held lands is eliminated, and equal access is gained by those without the "secret" environmental and social knowledge. The traditional allocation system, which is built on the recognition of natural variables, is replaced by a system organized to suit the demands of a capitalist economy.

Development goals of increasing production result in ecological deterioration. For example, in Senegal, 25,000 hectares put under irrigation for rice are now degraded, as inexperienced people quickly erected poorly built irrigation structures in order to satisfy a government requirement for establishing tenure. Polders constructed to control water flow are not flexible enough in times of drought. Polders also affect fishing, as

Risks of Genetically Modified Crops

The concerns over GM [genetically modified] crops are serious and the threats real. Every country has the sovereign right to take precautionary measures to address the risks involved. . . .

In the context of GM food aid, many stakeholders have underlined specific risks. Norway's Minister of International Development, for example, has said: "There might also be a probability of a higher risk when one is in a food crisis situation, consuming only one GMO [genetically modified organism] product over time".

The US government has often said that US citizens have been consuming GM foods for years and have never had any problems. However, Zambian scientists came to the conclusion that this argument is not valid in the African context: "While it is often said that GM maize is consumed by millions of Americans, it was noted that it is eaten in highly processed form and is not a staple food in the USA. In Zambia maize is the staple food and is usually the only carbohydrate source."

Many organizations in developing countries believe that populations fed with food aid, especially children, are particularly vulnerable due to malnutrition and lack of food, and that any potential danger presented by GM foods might increase when they are consumed by an immune-depressed population. According to the UK Chief Scientific Advisor Professor David King, forcing GM foods into Africa as food aid is "a massive human experiment".

Africa Center for Biosafety et al.,
GM Food Aid: Africa Denied Choice Once Again?
May 2004.

changes in the flow of the river and the displacement of water through polders affect fish breeding and feeding. The transition to a market economy ignores the nature of the Sahelian climate and soils and deprives traditional Marka groups of their ability to respond flexibly in times of environmental distress.

Introduction of transgenic crops into such regions will further accelerate the loss of indigenous knowledge and culture that make the traditional system sustainable. For example, [Ronald] Nigh and colleagues [writing in *Science*] have pointed out that characteristics of genetically altered grain could spread to local varieties favored by small-scale farmers and dilute the natural sustainability of these races.

Why GM Crops Will Not Work

In developing regions of the world, owners of large farms are much more likely to adopt genetically modified crops because they are better able to afford the seeds. However, small farms are often able to be more productive per unit of land than large farms, because small farms are more likely to be managed intensively. [Francesca Bray in *Scientific American* and Christian Castellanet and myself in the book *Participatory Action Research in Natural Resource Management*] give specific reasons why intensively managed farms may be more productive:

- Small farmers are more likely to plant various crops on the same field, plant multiple times during the year, and integrate crops, livestock, and even aquaculture, making more intensive use of space and time.

- Large farms are oriented toward large land enterprises such as cattle grazing or extensive grain monocultures, while small farmers emphasize labor and resource-intensive use of land.

- Farmers with large holdings are often more interested in land speculation.

- Small farmers are often more interested in sustainability, so that they can pass the farm on to at least some of their children.

- Small farms generally use family labor that is personally committed to the success of the farm, and large farms use relatively alienated hired labor.

- Because small farms have less land, small farmers often apply more labor per unit area.

- Small farms generally tend to use nonpurchased inputs like manure and compost, whereas large farms tend to use purchased inputs like agrochemicals.

- Small farmers may make more efficient use of irrigation.

- Large-scale farmers are less committed to management of other resources such as surrounding forest and streams, which are important for regional sustainability.

Conway argues that genetic engineering should be included in the list of factors that are important in intensification of agriculture in developing countries. However, [writing in *Bioscience*, David A.] Cleveland and colleagues suggest that incorporating folk varieties into the development of locally based agriculture may be a better approach, because farmer management of selection supports long-term yield stability that has been adapted to local conditions and cultural values. In contrast, genetically modified crops are engineered to perform well where agrochemicals are cheap and easily available, a situation that is not common in regions where hunger is a problem.

The Limits of Technology

Just because alternative agriculture cannot solve world hunger today, that does not mean that it should be ignored and that all hope be placed in biotechnology. Technologies by themselves are not enough.

[Conway quotes Professor Michael Lipton, an economist studying food and agriculture issues in developing countries, as stating] "There is a limit to technical cures for social pathologies. Too often the new technologies have been injected into communities with rapidly growing populations already dominated by excessive inequalities where, in the absence of countervailing policies, the powerful and the better-off have acquired the major share of the benefits. As a consequence, a high proportion, over 20 per cent, of the developing world's population is still poor and hungry."

It may be time to give equal resources to alternative approaches. Shouldn't we give a chance to agriculture that does not rely on genetic engineering? As Wes Jackson of the Land Institute likes to say, "Sustainable agriculture at this point in time is comparable to where flight was with the Wright Brothers in 1903."

The belief that genetic engineering can . . . relieve world hunger has made it difficult to realize that genetically modified crops have . . . widened the gap between rich and poor in developing countries. Reluctance to challenge such beliefs has led to massive investments in genetic engineering to the neglect of other more promising but less glamorous approaches. . . . In developing countries, new approaches could mean encouraging rediscovery of local crop varieties that are ecologically and culturally adapted to local conditions. Finally, small farmers in food-deprived countries could be encouraged to grow food for their families and neighbors instead of commodities to be sold abroad by the national government.

> *"Commercial livestock cloning could inundate the food supply with novel products that have not been safety tested."*

Cloned Animals Should Not Be Used for Food

Joseph Mendelson III

In the following viewpoint, Joseph Mendelson III opposes the use of cloned animals in the food production process and outlines the risks associated with this technology. He contends that using cloned animals to produce food jeopardizes both animal and human welfare. Furthermore, he maintains that studies conducted on cloned animals thus far have either shown grave defects with the animals or have not conclusively demonstrated the safety of clone-derived food products. Joseph Mendelson III is the co-founder and legal director of the Center for Food Safety.

As you read, consider the following questions:

1. According to Mendelson, what percentage of cloning attempts fail?

Joseph Mendelson III, "Initial Comments Concerning the Food and Drug Administration's Animal Cloning Risk Assessment," The Center for Food Safety, November 4, 2003. Reproduced by permission.

2. What examples does the author use to illustrate the different ways that cloning causes animals to suffer?

3. In Mendelson's opinion, what are several ways that cloning can degrade the food supply?

The widespread commercialization of cloned animals poses numerous issues that need to be further addressed prior to the completion of any risk assessment and conclusions concerning commercialization. These issues include animal welfare issues, in-depth edible product analysis, study of novel herd management issues that might arise because of cloned animal health and novel slaughter issues. . . .

Changing Humans' Relationship with Animals

The cloning of animals represents a fundamental change in our relationship with animals. The relationship changes human interaction with animals from an assistant in reproduction to a wholesale creator of genetic "replicas" of existing animals. The results of this relational change manifest themselves in the abhorrent animal suffering, a cruelty that will grow should cloning become a widespread commercial venture.

[Embryologist] Ian Wilmut and his team of scientists implanted 277 cloned sheep embryos in surrogate ewes, from which only thirteen pregnancies resulted and Dolly [the first mammal ever cloned] was the only successful birth. Even after several years of additional research and the development of new methods for extracting and transferring genetic material, well over 99% of all cloning attempts still fail. Even when nuclear transfers produce embryos that are successfully implanted in surrogates, only 3% to 5% of these pregnancies produce offspring that live to adulthood.

In one case, researchers at Texas A&M University set out to compare the development rates of cloned cattle derived from somatic and fetal cells. Only 17% of 322 adult SCNTs [somatic cell nuclear transfers] and 12% of 332 fetal cell nuclear transfers developed into embryos. Of these, 26 adult-cell-derived embryos and 32 fetal-cell-derived embryos were successfully implanted in surrogate mothers. After 40 days of pregnancy, six of the adult-cell-derived fetuses and three of the fetal-cell-derived fetuses survived. After 290 days of pregnancy, the experiment's only viable calf was born—a clone derived from an adult somatic cell. The project's 654 total nuclear cell transfers and 58 pregnancies had resulted in only one viable offspring. But even this meager success rate was tainted. "The cloned calf produced in this experiment possessed significant metabolic and cardiopulmonary abnormalities similar to those observed in previous studies," the researchers reported. In addition, the calf was born with diabetes mellitus and was found to be susceptible to severe immune-system deficiencies.

Inducing Animal Suffering

Cloned livestock that manage to survive birth tend to require more care than those sexually reproduced. Cloned calves, piglets, and lambs often require neonatal glucose infusions to treat hypoglycemia or oxygen treatments to offset hypoxia. Jonathan Hill, who has worked on cattle cloning at Cornell University, suspects that 25% to 50% of clones are born having been deprived of normal levels of oxygen. The neonatal condition of most clones is so poor, Rebecca Krisher, an animal reproduction specialist at Purdue University, says, "Almost all of these animals, if born on a farm without a vet hospital, . . . probably wouldn't survive."

The tremendous suffering of animal clones also impact their surrogate hosts. Most cloned livestock also exhibit a condition known as "large-offspring syndrome," which results in overly stressful deliveries for the surrogate mothers. Because of their large size, a higher than normal percentage of clones are delivered via cesarean section. In one documented cattle cloning project, three out of 12 surrogate mothers died during pregnancy.

Even the cloned animals that survive to be born are likely to suffer a wide range of health problems. One example is a sheep cloned by Ian Wilmut and his team, the same group who brought Dolly into the world. This much less heralded sheep, born not long after Dolly, had a malformed respiratory tract and was soon euthanized. In fact, such abnormalities are common. Late in 2002, scientists at the New Zealand government's AgResearch reported that 24% of the cloned calves born at the facility died between birth and weaning. This compares to a 5% mortality rate for non-cloned calves. Another 5% of cloned calves died after weaning, compared to 3% of sexually reproduced calves. One review of scientific literature, authored by executives at the commercial cloning lab Advanced Cell Technology, found that nearly 25% of cow, sheep, swine, and mouse clones showed severe developmental problems soon after birth. However, the vast majority of the studies considered for this review had follow-up periods of only a few weeks or months. Many later-developing health problems would not be reflected.

These results clearly indicate that cloning has a significant and overwhelming impact on the animals involved in the process. Consumers and the public have consistently rejected the animal suffering caused by cloning based upon moral grounds. . . .

Early Death in Cloned Animals

In addition to the animal welfare issues, data concerning the health of adult clone animals raises the specter of significant unresolved issues of food safety. Recent research shows that even clones seeming healthy at birth may not be as normal as they appear. Scientists at Tokyo's National Institute of Infectious Diseases found that cloned mice had significantly shorter life spans than normal mice. The research team raised 12 apparently healthy cloned mice and seven sexually reproduced mice in a controlled laboratory environment. At about 300 days after birth, the first cloned mouse died. Within 800 days of birth, 10 of the 12 clones had died, while six of the seven sexually reproduced mice were still thriving. Autopsies revealed that the clones died from a variety of maladies, including liver failure, pneumonia due to weak immune systems, and cancer.

Late-developing health problems are not confined to mouse clones. In fact, Dolly, often touted as livestock cloning's greatest success story, developed premature arthritis. Even more seriously, in February [2003] veterinarians at the Roslin Institute decided to euthanize Dolly after diagnosing her with a progressive lung disease. Dolly was only six years old. Researchers said that her normal life expectance would have been 11 or 12 years.

The most likely causes of clones' prenatal and postnatal defects are genetic abnormalities that arise during fetal development. Rudolf Jaenisch and colleagues at Massachusetts Institute of Technology's Whitehead Institute determined that cloned mice in their study had hundreds of improperly expressed genes. These resulted in a wide variety of abnormalities, ranging from the very subtle to the catastrophic. With so-called "imprinted genes," those that in a normal offspring only one copy—either from the mother or the father—is "switched on," Jaenisch found that nearly half "were incorrectly expressed." Though his experiments dealt only with cloned mice, Jaenisch concluded that genetic abnormalities were most likely responsible for the dismal success rates of cattle, sheep, and swine cloning efforts. "There is no reason in the world to assume that any other mammal . . . would be different from mice," he said. Davor Solter of Germany's Max Planck Insti

Ethics Advisory Committee on Animal Cloning Needed

[Sixty-three percent] of Americans . . . want the government to factor in ethical considerations when making a decision on animal cloning. It is therefore essential that the federal government establish an ethics committee to publicly discuss and advise the FDA [Food and Drug Administration] and Health and Human Services (FDA's parent agency) on such matters *before* animals are allowed to be commercially cloned for food.

Given the severity of the animal health problems associated with cloning, and the magnitude of ethical qualms Americans have with using the technology, there is both a pressing need and an overwhelming demand for the government to establish a proper regulatory framework to oversee animal cloning, one that takes into consideration both ethics and science. An advisory committee, mirroring the Health and Human Services' Secretary's Advisory Committee on Genetics, Health, and Society, which serves as a public forum for deliberations on the broad societal issues raised by the development and use of genetic technologies in humans, must be established to deliberate both publicly and officially the ethical challenges presented by animal cloning.

American Anti-Vivisection Society,
December 2006. www.EndAnimalCloning.org.

tute for Immunobiology says it is likely that few if any clones are completely free of genetic abnormalities. "Whether the clone dies next day or next year depends on how badly it misses," he said.

Differences of Cloned Animals

In normally reproduced animals, a methylation switches certain genes off as the animal matures and the functions encoded by those genes are no longer necessary. Methylation also plays a role in the proper expression of imprinted genes. Because SCNT cloning uses genetic material from mature cells, the methylation pattern in these clones is often quite different than in animals that develop as normal embryos. While scientists try to "reprogram" the adult genetic material to act as if it were embryonic DNA, a group of South Korean scientists who studied SCNT cloned cow embryos detected no indications of methylation; they found this resulted in unusual patterns of genetic imprinting. The research team concluded that this incomplete genetic reprogramming could be one reason for the high failure rate of animal cloning.

A second study, presented in the June 2001 issue of *Genesis*, also showed abnormal methylation in clones, leading to unpredictable health problems, including overgrown placentas, increased body weight, and respiratory, blood or immune system problems. "No matter what you do, cloning changes these methylation flags," said one scientist. Jaenisch and his colleagues at the Whitehead Institute concluded that improper methylation caused the abnormalities they found with imprinted genes in their cloned mice. "Even apparently normal clones have an abnormal regulation of many genes," Jaenisch said. "Completely normal clones may be the exception." In fact, improper methylation may be cloning's fatal flaw. Writing in *Science*, Wilmut and Jaenisch state that there is no way now or for the foreseeable future for scientists to detect whether these reprogramming errors have occurred.

In August of 2003 researchers at the University of Connecticut report the sudden death of three cloned adult pigs. The reasons associated with these animal deaths remain unresolved. Nonetheless, the scientists suspect it is the result of abnormal gene regulation caused by methylation issues.

Unhealthy Clones, Unhealthy Food

Many scientists are concerned that these subtle and not-so-subtle "imprinting errors" raise as yet unresolved safety issues concerning the food products from cloned livestock. Ian Wilmut has said that commercial production of meat and dairy products from cloned animals should not begin until large-scale, controlled trials have been conducted. Cloners now working on dairy production say they are comparing the milk from their clones with natural milk, but Wilmut told the magazine *New Scientist* that study of cloned animals should look not only at milk, but also at the animals' health profiles and life spans. Wilmut warned that even small imbalances in an animal's hormone, protein, and fat levels could compromise the quality and safety of meat and milk.

While Infigen and other cloning companies have already proclaimed the safety of their food products, scientists have yet to complete necessary studies. The NAS' [National Academy of Sciences] August 2002 report on animal biotechnology notes that scant research on the safety of meat and milk from embryo-derived clones exists. As for SCNT cloning, food safety issues are even less clear, as the NAS notes:

> The cloning of animals from somatic cells is more recent. Limited sample size, health and production data, and rapidly changing cloning protocols make it difficult to draw conclusions regarding the safety of milk, meat, or other products from individuals that are themselves somatic cell cloned individuals.

Some scientists warn that abnormal gene-expression, which likely causes the health problems of clones, is likely to also affect the meat and milk of cloned livestock. The NAS notes that studies to confirm or refute this have not been done: "There are to date no published ... comparative analytical data assessing the composition of meat and milk products of somatic cell clones, their offspring, and conventionally bred animals." FDA's reliance on one study concerning milk derived from cloned animals and the no meat studies does little to alter the NAS' finding that the science necessary to adequately assess risks does not yet exist. Similarly, FDA cannot point to studies that adequately assess whether abnormal gene-expression creates inherited traits in cloned animals' progeny.

Additional food safety concerns stem from the high failure rates of cloning pregnancies and the typical sickly nature of newborn clones. Scientists often infuse the surrogate mothers of cloned livestock with massive doses of hormones to improve the odds that the cloned embryos will implant in the surrogates' uteruses. While the clones are typically the genetic offspring of highly prized parents, the surrogate mothers hold no such intrinsic value. Many surrogate mothers are destined for slaughterhouses soon after giving birth, opening an avenue for large amounts of veterinary pharmaceuticals to enter the human food supply. The clones themselves, often born with severely compromised immune systems, frequently receive massive doses of antibiotics and other medications. Commercialization of cloning would almost certainly increase levels of veterinary hormones and antibiotics in the human food supply.

Commercialization of cloned livestock for food production could also increase the incidence of food-borne illnesses, such as *E. coli* infections, resulting from slaughter of such animals. According to the NAS study:

> Because stress from [the] developmental problems [of cloned livestock] might result in shedding of pathogens in fecal material, resulting in a higher load of undesirable microbes on the carcass, the food safety of products, especially such as veal, from young somatic cell cloned animals might indirectly present a . . . concern. . . .

Reducing Genetic Diversity

Finally, the allowance of commercialized cloning may broadly affect the overall health of the U.S. farm animal population by further eroding genetic diversity. Modern livestock breeding techniques have already reduced the genetic diversity of many populations of farm animals. Over 90% of U.S. dairy cows are the Holstein variety. Eight of the 15 breeds of swine raised in the United States in the middle of the 20th century no longer exist. Similarly, only five breeds comprise nearly the entire U.S. poultry flock, and almost all white eggs come from white leghorns. Large-scale commercial cloning of animals would further erode livestock diversity. Entire herds and flocks could share a single genome. While breeders would aim to clone animals with desirable genetic characteristics, genetic weaknesses would inevitably be passed along as well. Herds of genetically identical animals would likely be highly susceptible to communicable diseases and environmental hazards. One NAS scientist has warned that allowing cloning in livestock production could lead to "genetic bottlenecks" that dilute diversity and leave farms vulnerable to epidemic disease. According to the U.K. Farm Animal Welfare Council,

> [T]he potential of introducing deleterious genes ... must not be forgotten. Furthermore, any tendency to lose genetic diversity may make it difficult or even impossible to reverse the effect of such deleterious genes once recognised. This might result in an increased risk of genetic abnormalities, susceptibility to disease and other welfare consequences. We do not believe that control of these problems should be left to the industry but rather that statutory regulation is required.

For consumers, commercial livestock cloning could inundate the food supply with novel products that have not been safety tested and have raised safety concerns among some of the leading scientists in the cloning field. For farm animals, the spread of cloning is likely to bring genetic defects, premature aging, and widespread suffering.

> "[The U.S. Food and Drug Administration] concluded that meat and milk from cattle, swine, and goat clones would be as safe as food we eat from those species now."

Cloned Animals Are Safe to Use for Food

Siobhan DeLancey, Larisa Rudenko, and John Matheson

In the following viewpoint, Siobhan DeLancey, Larisa Rudenko, and John Matheson state that it is safe and beneficial to introduce cloned animals into the food production supply chain. The authors contend that cloning is not unlike previously employed reproduction techniques, such as in vitro *fertilization, and generally offers the same benefits and limited risks. In addition, they state that cloning offers farmers the ability to better control the traits of animals in their herds, which in turn provides them with the opportunity to increase the overall quality of their product. Finally, they recount the rigorous testing that has been carried out on clones to prove these animals and their offspring are safe. Siobhan DeLancey is a consumer safety officer for the Food and Drug Administration (FDA). Larisa Rudenko is a senior advisor for biotechnology at the Center for Veterinary Medi-*

Siobhan DeLancey, Larisa Rudenko, and John Matheson, "A Primer on Cloning and Its Use in Livestock Operations," *FDA Veterinarian*, vol. 21, no. 5, 2006, pp. 6–9.

cine within the FDA. John Matheson is a senior regulatory review scientist at the Office of Surveillance and Compliance within the FDA.

As you read, consider the following questions:

1. According to the authors, are there any differences between the complications associated with natural or assisted reproductive practices and cloning?
2. Why do DeLancey, Rudenko, and Matheson state that cloning can help farmers improve the quality of their herds?
3. What is the purpose of animal clones in the dairy and meat trades, according to the authors?

Imagine the perfect dairy cow. For eight years she has gotten pregnant on the first try, given birth easily, and produced gallon upon gallon of the best milk. Even when others in the herd got sick, she stayed healthy. She is ideally suited to the climate in which she lives. The farmer has depended on this cow and her daughters in lean times to carry the farm through, but now she is at the end of her reproductive life.

Although the farmer may have this cow's daughters to carry on the line, he also has another alternative: copying her. Biological copying is referred to as cloning. By cloning his prize cow, breeding the clones, and keeping their offspring, the farmer can introduce the natural positive characteristics into the herd quickly. It would take several more years to achieve these same improvements by conventional breeding.

Farmers can also clone animals to produce more uniform quality meat. Take, for example, a male pig (boar) who time after time sires piglets that mature quickly and provide lean meat. If a farmer has several of these boars he could quickly produce an entire herd with consistent, high quality meat.

Researchers have been cloning livestock since 1996. In 2001, when it became apparent that cloning could become a commercial venture, the Food and Drug Administration's (FDA) Center for Veterinary Medicine (CVM) asked that food from clones and their offspring be voluntarily kept out of the food chain. FDA then began an intensive evaluation that included examining the safety of food from these animals.

Traditional Mating Is Rare

Cloning is a complex process that lets one exactly copy the genetic, or inherited, traits of an animal (the donor). Livestock species that scientists have successfully cloned are cattle, pigs, sheep, and goats. Scientists have also cloned mice, rats, rabbits, cats, mules, horses, and one dog. Chickens and other poultry have not been cloned.

Most people think of livestock breeding taking place through traditional mating, in which males and females physically get together to reproduce. In fact, this type of mating is not often the case.

Traditional mating is not that efficient, if the goal is to produce as many offspring as possible. For example, a male has enough sperm to produce many more offspring than would be possible by traditional mating. Traditional mating also has certain risks: one or both of the animals may be injured in the process of mating. The female may be hurt by the male because he is often so much larger, or an unwilling female may injure the male. There is also a risk of infection or transmission of venereal disease during traditional mating.

Because of these factors, many farmers use assisted reproductive technologies for breeding. These include artificial insemination, embryo transfer, and *in vitro* fertilization. Artificial insemination was first documented in the breeding of horses in the 14th century. The first successful embryo transfer of a cow was in 1951, and the first *in vitro* fertilization (IVF)-derived animal was a rabbit born in 1959. Livestock production in the United States now uses all these methods regularly. For example, most dairy farms don't have bulls, so more than 70% of the Holstein cows bred in the United States are artificially inseminated. The frozen semen can come from a bull many miles, or even many states, away.

An Advanced Reproductive Technology

Cloning is a more advanced form of these assisted reproductive technologies. Much of the public perception of cloning likely comes from science fiction books and movies. Some people incorrectly believe that clones spring forth fully formed, or are grown in test tubes. This is just not the case. Clones are born just like other animals. They are similar to identical twins, only born at different times. Just as twins share the same DNA, clones have the same genes as the donor animal. A clone is not a mutant, nor is it a weaker version of the original animal. It's just a copy.

In all of the other assisted reproductive technologies, the male and female parents each contribute half of their genes to their offspring. Farmers have worked for years to choose animals with the best traits and breed them together, which increases the chance these good traits will be passed on and become more common in livestock herds. Even though farmers have been able to improve their herds over time, they still can't absolutely predict the characteristics of the offspring, not even their sex. Cloning gives the farmer complete control over the offspring's inherited traits. Thus, a farmer who clones an especially desirable, but aging or injured animal knows in advance that the clone will have the genetic potential to be an especially good, younger animal. He can then use that animal to further reproduce by traditional mating or other assisted breeding.

Like *In Vitro* Fertilization

Most cloning today uses a process called somatic cell nuclear transfer (SCNT). Just as with *in vitro* fertilization, scientists take an immature egg from a female animal (often from ovaries obtained at the slaughter-house). But instead of combining it with sperm, they remove the nucleus (which contains the egg's genes). This leaves behind the other components necessary for an embryo to develop. Scientists then add the nucleus containing the desirable traits from the animal the farmer wishes to copy. After a few other steps, the donor nucleus and egg fuse, start dividing, and an embryo begins to form. The embryo is then implanted in the uterus of a surrogate dam (again the same as with *in vitro* fertilization), which carries it to term. ("Dam" is a term that livestock breeders use to refer to the female parent of an animal). The clone is delivered just like any other baby animal.

There are no complications that are unique to cloning. These problems are also seen in animals born from natural mating or assisted reproductive technologies. They seem to happen more often in clones for a number of reasons that probably have to do with parts of the procedure that occur outside the body. The embryo may fail to develop properly during the *in vitro* stage or early on after transfer to the surrogate and may be flushed out of the uterus. If it does develop, the embryo may not implant properly into the uterus of the surrogate dam. Alternatively, the placenta may not form properly, and the developing animal won't get the nourishment it needs.

Large Offspring Syndrome (LOS) is seen in pregnancies of cattle and sheep that come from both assisted reproductive technologies and cloning. With LOS, the fetus grows too large in the uterus, making problems for the animal and its surrogate dam. LOS has not been observed in goats and swine.

As a group, livestock clones tend to have more health problems at birth, and may die more often right after birth than conventionally bred animals. If clones survive the first few days after birth, they seem to become just as healthy and strong as other animals of the same age. By the time clones are young adults, it's not possible to tell them apart from other animals of the same age, even if you conduct a detailed examination. Scientists at FDA and research institutions have looked at blood work for clones that's similar to what people get when they have physicals. These results show that the clones are perfectly healthy, and walk, wean, grow, mature, and behave just like conventional animals.

Cloning Makes Food Better

The main use of clones is to produce breeding stock, not food. Clones allow farmers to upgrade the overall quality of their herds by providing more copies of the best animals in the herd. These animals are then used for conventional breeding, and the sexually reproduced offspring become the food-producing animals. Just as farmers wouldn't use their best conventionally bred breeding animals as sources of food, they are equally unlikely to do so for clones.

Some examples of desirable characteristics in livestock that breeders might want in their herds include the following:

- Disease resistance: Sick animals are expensive for farmers. Veterinary bills add up, and unhealthy animals don't produce as much meat or milk. A herd that is resistant to disease is extremely valuable because it doesn't lose any production time to illness, and doesn't cost the farmer extra money for veterinary treatment.

- Suitability to climate: Different types of livestock grow well in different climates. Some of this is natural and some results from selective breeding. For instance, Brahma cattle can cope with the heat and humidity of weather in the southwestern United States, but they often do not produce very high grades of meat. Cloning could allow breeders to select those cattle that can produce high quality meat or milk and thrive in extreme climates and use them to breed more cattle to be used for food production. Similarly, pork production

Moral Concerns About Cloning Do Not Justify Government Intervention

The ethical concerns [related to cloning animals for food] are primarily moral considerations that legitimately could influence actions taken by individual breeders, producers, and consumers, but not legitimately be used to argue for government intervention. Even the FDA [Food and Drug Administration] agrees with this point. In its proposed risk management plan, the agency states: "The Draft Risk Assessment is strictly a science-based evaluation of animal health and food consumption risks, and the Proposed Risk Management Plan and Draft Guidance for Industry do not address any ethical or other non-science based concerns regarding animal cloning."

Most ethical objections to cloning and genetic engineering in general come from a fear of the unknown consequences of such technology, a religious or moral objection to tampering with natural reproduction, and/or a concern for preventing cruelty to animals. While all these concerns hold legitimate moral sway with various portions of the population, they are not grounds for government action. We live in a pluralist society and those who disagree on religious or moral grounds with cloning should be free to speak out, boycott, or not participate in the objectionable activity, but those who do not object should be equally free to participate in producing food from clones and/or eating it.

Sigrid Fry-Revere, "Cloned Food 101,"
Cato-at-Liberty, December 29, 2006.

has traditionally been centered in the eastern United States, but is moving to different regions of the United

States (e.g., Utah). Cloning could allow breeders to select those pigs that naturally do well in the new climate, and use them to breed more pigs to be used for food production.

- Quality body type: Farmers naturally want an animal whose body is well suited to its production function. For example, a dairy cow should have a large, well-attached udder so that she can produce lots of milk. She should also be able to carry and deliver calves easily. For animals that produce meat, farmers breed for strong, heavy-muscled, quick-maturing animals that will yield high quality meat in the shortest time possible. The most desirable bulls produce offspring that are relatively small at birth (so that they are easier for the female to carry and deliver), but that grow rapidly and are healthy after birth.

- Fertility: Quality dairy cows should be very fertile, because a cow that doesn't get pregnant and bear calves won't produce milk. Male fertility is just as important as that of the female. The more sperm he can produce, the more females a bull can inseminate, and the more animals will be born. Beef cattle or other meat-producing animals such as pigs need to have high fertility rates in order to replace animals that are sent to slaughter. Cloning allows farmers and breeders to clone those animals with high fertility rates so that they could bear offspring that would also tend to be very fertile.

- Market preference: Farmers or ranchers may also want to breed livestock to meet the changing tastes of consumers. The traits the producers are looking for include leanness, tenderness, color, and size of various cuts. Preferences also vary by culture, and cloning may help tailor products to the preferences of various international markets and ethnic groups.

How does cloning help get these characteristics into the herd more quickly? As we've previously said, cloning allows the breeder to increase the number of breeding animals available to make the actual food production animals. So, if a producer wanted to introduce disease resistance into a herd rapidly, cloning could be used to produce a number of breeding animals that carry the gene for disease resistance, rather than just one. Likewise, if a breeder wants to pass on the genes of a female animal, cloning could result in multiples of that female to breed, rather than just one.

Studies Show Clone-Derived Food to Be Safe

It's important to remember that the purpose of clones is for breeding, not eating. Dairy, beef, or pork clones will make up a tiny fraction of the total number of food producing animals in the United States. Instead, their offspring will be the animals actually producing meat or milk for the food supply.

Dairy clones will produce milk after they give birth, and the dairy farmers will want to be able to drink that milk or put it in the food supply. Once clones used for breeding meat-producing animals can no longer reproduce, their breeders will also want to be able to put them into the food supply.

In order to determine whether there would be any risk involved in eating meat or milk from clones or their offspring, in 1999 FDA asked the National Academy of Sciences (NAS) to identify science-based concerns associated with animal biotechnology, including cloning. The NAS gathered an independent group of top, peer-selected scientists from across the country to conduct this study. The scientists delivered their report in the fall of 2002. That report stated that theoretically there were no concerns for the safety of meat or milk from clones. On the other hand, the report expressed a low level of concern due to a lack of information on the clones at that time, and not for any specific scientific reasons. The report also stated that the meat and milk from the offspring of clones posed no unique food safety concerns.

Meanwhile, FDA itself began the most comprehensive examination of the health of livestock clones that has been conducted. The evaluation has taken more than four years. This examination formed the basis of a Draft Risk Assessment to determine whether cloning posed a risk to animal health or to humans eating food from clones or their offspring. FDA conducted a thorough search of the scientific literature on clones, and identified hundreds of peer-reviewed scientific journal articles, which it then reviewed. They were also able to obtain health records and blood samples from almost all of the cattle clones that have been produced in the United States and data from clones produced in other countries. FDA compared these health records, and the independently analyzed blood results with similar samples from conventional animals of the same age and breed that were raised on the same farms.

After reviewing all this information, FDA found that it could not tell a healthy clone from a healthy conventionally bred animal. All of the blood values, overall health records, and behaviors were in the same range for clones and conventional animals of the same breed raised on the same farms. FDA also saw that milk from dairy clones does not differ significantly in composition from milk from conventionally bred animals.

In the Draft Risk Assessment, FDA concluded that meat and milk from cattle, swine, and goat clones would be as safe as food we eat from those species now. It did not have enough information to make a decision on the safety of food from sheep clones.

For another study similar to the one conducted on cow clones, the Agency also evaluated the health of offspring sexually derived from swine clones, as well as the composition of their meat. After reviewing this very large data set, the Agency concluded that all of the blood values, overall health records, and meat composition profiles of the progeny of clones were in the same range as for very closely genetically related conventionally bred swine. Based on these results, other studies from scientific journals, and our understanding of the biological processes involved in cloning, the Agency agreed with NAS that food from the sexually reproduced offspring of clones is as safe as food that we eat every day. These offspring animals will produce almost all of the food from the overall cloning/ breeding process.

Periodical Bibliography

The following articles have been selected to supplement the diverse views presented in this chapter.

Mark Anslow	"10 Reasons Why GM Won't Feed the World," *Ecologist*, January 3, 2008. www.theecologist.org.
Oliver Broudy	"Guess What's Coming to Dinner," *Men's Health*, November 2006.
Verlyn Klinkenborg	"Closing the Barn Door After the Cows Have Gotten Out," *New York Times*, January 23, 2008.
Sean McDonagh	"Genetic Engineering Is Not the Answer," *America*, May 2, 2005.
Henry I. Miller	"Food from Cloned Animals Is Part of Our Brave New World," *Trends in Biotechnology*, May 2007.
John Nichols	"The World Food Crisis," *Nation*, May 12, 2008.
Robert Paarlberg	"From the Green Revolution to the Gene Revolution," *Environment*, January/February 2005.
Jeffrey M. Smith	"Frankenstein Peas," *Ecologist*, April 2006.
Paul Spackman	"Can GM Crops End Food Supply Shortage Fears?" *Farmer's Weekly*, October 26, 2007.
Colin Tudge	"Profits Won't Feed the World," *New Statesman*, November 10, 2003.
Starre Vartan	"Ah-tchoo!" *E-The Environmental Magazine*, November/December 2006.

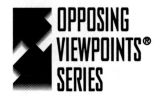
**OPPOSING
VIEWPOINTS®
SERIES**

How Should Genetic Engineering Technology Be Regulated?

Chapter Preface

Labeling genetically modified (GM) foods in the United States has been a voluntary process since 1992. Current U.S. Food and Drug Administration guidelines require no labeling or additional safety testing on genetically modified foods as long as the product is found to be "substantially equivalent" to its nonmodified counterpart. However, there have been documented cases where the GM product has had a detrimental impact on consumers.

Showa Denko K. K., a chemical engineering firm based in Tokyo, Japan, has produced many food supplements over the years, including the essential amino acid tryptophan, which is necessary for protein biosynthesis. Tryptophan, which is found in most protein-rich foods, is often manufactured through the process of fermentation. Large quantities of bacteria are grown in vats, and then the tryptophan is extracted from the bacteria.

In 1987, in an effort to increase tryptophan production, the company opted to use genetically engineered bacteria. Inserting several genes into the bacteria resulted in higher levels of already present enzymes and allowed for enzymes that are not normally found in the bacteria. As the company hoped, the modifications affected the bacteria's metabolism, causing them to produce tryptophan much more efficiently. By 1988, the genetically engineered bacteria were being used for the commercial production of tryptophan and were also being sold in the United States. Showa Denko K. K. was allowed to sell their genetically engineered product in the States because the company had been producing tryptophan from nongenetically engineered bacteria for many years without ill effect. In this instance, however, within a few months, thirty-seven people died from eating the modified bacteria and more than fifteen hundred were permanently disabled. Due to a lack of labeling, it was impossible to distinguish the genetically modified tryptophan from the nonmodified variety, and therefore it took several months to discover that it was indeed the genetically engineered tryptophan that caused the problem.

The genetically engineered tryptophan was found to contain highly toxic contaminants that were created when the compromised bacteria produced excessive tryptophan levels. The toxins caused the consumers to suffer eosinophilia myalgia syndrome (EMS), a condition resulting in paralysis, neurological problems, heart conditions, swelling and cracking of the skin, and in some cases, death. However, scientists were never able to study the defective tryptophan. Showa Denko K. K. destroyed all contaminated bacteria when the safety issues were brought to light. The company paid out more than two billion dollars in damages.

Cases such as this make the oversight of genetically engineered foods and food supplements a controversial issue. This is just one of the topics addressed in the following chapter. Other viewpoints in the chapter deal with gene patenting and the safeguarding of personal genetic information—topics that all revolve around the question of how much regulation is needed to ensure that genetic engineering benefits rather than harms consumers.

> "Banning [gene] patents risks shutting down a large part of the [biotech] industry and creating a major roadblock to progress in patient care and food."

Gene Patenting Should Be Allowed

Geoffrey M. Karny

In the following viewpoint, Geoffrey M. Karny argues that gene patents advance technological discovery in the field of biomedicine. He contends that patents are necessary because they provide corporations with the incentive to invest in genetic research. Karny states that DNA sequences isolated in gene research are unique inventions and therefore are legally patentable. Geoffrey M. Karny is a partner at the Washington, D.C.–based law firm Baker & Daniels.

As you read, consider the following questions:

1. According to a Tufts University study cited by the author, how much money does it cost to bring a new drug to market?

Geoffrey M. Karny, "In Defense of Gene Patenting: The Principles of Our Patent System Are Sound and Bring Immense Benefits," *Genetic Engineering & Biotechnology News*, vol. 27, no. 7, April 1, 2007. Republished with permission of *Genetic Engineering & Biotechnology News*, conveyed through Copyright Clearance Center, Inc.

2. How do patents protect the public, in Karny's view?

3. For what reasons do patent owners want their inventions patented, according to the author?

Gene patenting has been under attack for several years. Various academics have been leading the charge, closely followed by groups that perceive their professional interests to be threatened.

Now science fiction novelist Michael Crichton has jumped on the bandwagon. In his book *Next*, Crichton brings forth a host of biotech bad guys who represent virtually every stereotype imaginable. They include a greedy venture capitalist, dishonest and hypocritical scientists, a body-part-selling pathologist, and the obligatory sleazy lawyer.

Gene patenting is one of several biotech hot-button issues that run through the novel. In fact, Crichton even included an appendix in which he argues against gene patenting. It is the usual suspects—nobody should own our genes because they exist in nature, and gene patents are bad public policy because they suppress research and hurt patient care.

One is tempted to dismiss the novel, hoping that its poor reviews will limit the number of readers and, therefore, the dissemination of misinformation.

Unfortunately, the biotech industry cannot be complacent. Congressmen Xavier Becerra (D-Calif.) and David Weldon (R-Fla.) introduced a bill (H.R.977) to prospectively ban gene patents. The key provision states, "Notwithstanding any other provision of law, no patent may be obtained for a nucleotide sequence, or its functions or correlations, or the naturally occurring products it specifies." Congressman Becerra's introductory remarks make many of the same arguments that Crichton does.

Therefore, it is necessary to review, once again, the reasons why patents on genes are proper under U.S. patent law and why they represent wise social policy.

Patents Fund the Biotech Industry

Gene patents, more specifically patent claims to nucleotide sequences, such as genes, plasmids, and probes, are fundamental and critical to the biotech industry. They are the foundation of the industry. Such claims protect therapeutic proteins, like human insulin; Mabs[1], like Herceptin® [used to treat breast cancer]; transgenic plants, like insect-resistant corn; and diagnostic probes for genetic diseases, which are the foundation for personalized medicine. Banning such patents risks shutting down a large part of the industry and creating a major roadblock to progress in patient care and food production.

Inventions do not move from the laboratory to the marketplace without a huge investment of money, time, and effort. A Tufts University study has found that it takes over $800 million to bring a new drug to market. The author is not aware of similar studies for transgenic plants or gene-based diagnostics, but the cost must be substantial, even if less than for drugs.

For diagnostics in particular, critics have argued that it is a relatively quick and straightforward process for a laboratory to develop a molecular diagnostic once a particular disease-associated gene has been identified in the scientific literature. However, an examination of financial disclosure documents of some molecular diagnostic companies indicate that this is not the case.

For example, the prospectus for [genetic research firm] Genomic Health's IPO [initial public offering, issued to outline a company's mission when it offers its stock for sale to the public], dated September 8, 2005, states that the company would use $20 million of the proceeds to fund R&D [research and development]. [Research company] Third Wave's 10-K [annual report filed with the Securities and Exchange Com-

1. Mabs, or monocloral antibodies, are proteins produced by scientists in a laboratory from a single parent cell and used in biological therapies to treat illnesses such as cancer.

mission summarizing a company's financial performance] for 2005, the latest available, states that it spent $8.4 million for R&D for that year. These amounts would cover several products, but clearly a substantial amount of money is involved. Quite simply, this investment will not happen if, after it is done, a competitor can get a free ride on the pioneer's efforts and knock-off the product.

Patents Protect Inventors and the Public

The [U.S.] Constitution provides for patents. The founders recognized that it takes time, money, and effort to develop an invention to the point where it can benefit humankind. Thus, they authorized Congress to provide inventors with the right to exclude others from the invention for a limited period of time. Thus, a patent is a limited property right. It is not a reward. It is also not a monopoly, even though the right extends to a class of things, because a monopoly is defined by market power. As many a disappointed inventor well knows, having a patent is no guarantee of commercial success. Quite simply, a patent is granted to provide the inventor and/or his company or investors the incentive to undertake the costly and risky process of further development and commercialization. They will do so because they can charge enough for the product to recover their investment.

In return, the public gets the invention, but not for free. What it gets for free is the new technical knowledge to build on because the patent must disclose how to make and how to use the invention in terms that a person skilled in that technology can understand. And, after the patent expires, the public even gets the invention for free.

The public is protected because the patent statute permits no more than the actual contribution made by the inventor to be the subject of the limited property right. The invention must be novel, that is, not disclosed in any printed document found anywhere in the world or publicly known or used in the U.S. Thus, the law recognizes the basic fact that the inven-

Media Misunderstanding

Although gene patenting policy may be clear to scientists, companies, and many lawmakers, it isn't so clear to the public—and sometimes to the media. And that's why even just talking about the issue can cause panic—as it did in the stock market in April [2000] when investors and the media misinterpreted President [Bill] Clinton and British Prime Minister Tony Blair's comments suggesting that the human genome should be public property. "On the patent thing, you know, Tony Blair and I crashed the market there for a day, and I didn't mean to," Clinton said on April 5 [2000] following the joint statement he made with Blair on gene-based patents. Clinton and Blair were actually endorsing, not questioning, the trademark office's gene patenting policy. The media, however, misunderstood their position, and shareholders lost millions of dollars when their stocks plummeted.

Megan Lisagor, National Journal, *July 15, 2000.*

tor created something that did not exist before. The invention must be useful. The invention must not be obvious; that is, the novelty should not be a trivial one that any person of routine skill in the technology could have envisioned. The invention must be described in a manner to enable other people skilled in that technology to make and use it. This permits others in the field to build on the new knowledge. Finally, the invention must be clearly claimed so that the public knows the scope of the limited property right.

Making DNA Sequences Useful

Crichton and other critics often ask, "How can anyone own my genes?" The answer is that they cannot. What someone can "own" is a DNA sequence that he or she was the first to isolate and that is useful. Similarly, a person who discovers a new function of a known DNA sequence, such as its previously unknown association with a particular disease, can patent a method of using the isolated sequence to detect susceptibility to that disease. Isolated DNA sequences do not occur in nature. They are new.

Claiming them as isolated sequences is not "mere word play" as asserted by Congressman Becerra in his remarks. Rather, the language reflects the critical fact that, but for the actions of the inventor, the invention would not exist. The gene for human Factor VIII doesn't do a hemophiliac any good when it is in somebody else's genome. It is only useful when someone isolates it and a company spends time and money to bring human Factor VIII to the market. Since isolated DNA sequences do not occur in nature, they are not natural products. By patenting them, the inventor takes nothing from the public.

Myths Spun by Critics of Gene Patents

The critics say that gene patents are bad social policy—they hinder research, raise costs, and limit patient access to care.

Academic researchers believe that scientific advancement occurs through the publication of research results. Society agrees that research is valuable and encourages it through billions of dollars of taxpayer-funded grants. However, this culture of information-sharing and government grants appears to have created a culture of entitlement where the property rights of others, specifically patent rights, are expected to be freely available in the name of research.

As with any human activity, even one as important as scientific research, there have to be limits. Respecting the patent rights of others has to be one of those limits if society is going to gain the benefits of the patent system.

As a practical matter, however, academic scientists who ignore patent rights have little to fear. The vast majority of patent owners simply do not want the adverse publicity of suing scientists and their universities, and the economic recovery is seldom worth the effort and money spent. They want patents in order to exclude competitors, trade them for needed technology, or raise money from investors.

The often-cited case of *Madey v. Duke University*, where a former Duke University professor sued the university for infringement of patents that he owned, is an aberration. The university had forced Madey out of his position as a laboratory director, and he responded with a powerful weapon that he had at hand—a patent-infringement suit.

More importantly, the fact that Duke was found to have infringed his patents goes to a fundamental aspect of the patent law. The law recognizes a limited research exemption from infringement. This exemption is limited to an examination of the patented invention; that is, research on the invention. This is completely consistent with the policy underlying the patent law of encouraging others to build upon the knowledge disclosed in the patent, including developing improvements or "inventing around" the patent.

This is quite different from using the patented invention in research. Simply because an organization is a nonprofit entity and/or engaged in a noble enterprise like scientific research does not mean that the organization or its employees have the right to infringe the patents of others. A patented reagent may cost more, but that is simply a cost of engaging in the activity, like any other cost.

Critics have also charged that patents raise costs to patients and/or limit patient access to medical care. One cited study is [Mildred K. Cho et al., *Journal of Molecular Diagnostics*, 2003]. The article reports the results of a telephone survey of 211 directors of laboratories that do molecular diagnostic testing. Of 122 respondents, 25% reported discontinuing performing patented genetic tests, and 53% stated they did not develop new tests because of patents.

However, a closer examination of the article shows that the respondents simply did not want to pay to license the patented tests. One of the respondents even acknowledged this by stating, "People shouldn't be complaining that they can't run tests. They should just pay." Access to patented technology is a cost of doing business. Facilities and reagents are not free, and employees do not work for free. Why should new technology be free? The tests are available. It's just a question of cost.

Benefits of the Patent System

In the noise and misinformation about gene patents, basic, common-sense principles are lost. These principles have supported the patent system for over 200 years and have contributed to the technological greatness of this nation and to the benefits that technology brings to humankind. They bear repeating. The inventor brings something new to the world. The patent provides the incentive to bring it to market. And new biomedical and agricultural products improve the human condition.

Crichton and the other antigene patent folks love to talk about mouse traps. They have no problem with patenting better mouse traps. But society will have a problem if they get their way. We will have plenty of mouse traps but far fewer new drugs and diagnostics and far less food.

"It is time that [Congress] as a legislative body put an end to this practice [of patenting genes]."

Gene Patenting Should Be Banned

Xavier Becerra

In the following viewpoint, Democratic congressman Xavier Becerra from California argues that gene patenting should be banned. He contends that gene patenting harms society and hinders scientific advances because of all the restrictions and fees imposed on individuals wishing to use patented gene sequences in research or treatment. Additionally, Becerra argues that genes are not patentable because they are products of nature, not human invention. Xavier Becerra has been a member of the U.S. House of Representatives since 1992.

As you read, consider the following questions:

1. What are the five implications of gene patenting, according to Becerra?
2. What does the author say is the "analogous equivalent" of patenting a gene?

Xavier Becerra, "On the Introduction of the Genomic Research and Accessibility Act," speech before U.S. House of Representatives, February 9, 2007.

3. According to Becerra, what effects do patents on breast cancer genes have on a woman with breast cancer and her doctor?

I rise [to speak] today with the hope of fixing what I believe to be a regulatory mistake—a mistake that at first glance may seem minor in scope, but upon further examination has dramatic, costly and harmful implications for every American.

I speak of the practice of gene patenting, where private corporations, universities and even the federal government are granted a monopoly by the United States Patent and Trademark Office on significant sections of the human genome.

It is my belief that this practice is wrong, ill-conceived and stunts scientific advancement. And it is for this reason that today I introduce the Genomic Research and Accessibility Act to put an immediate end to this practice.

Fifty-four years ago this month [February 2007] [American molecular biologist] James Watson and [English molecular biologist] Francis Crick discovered the structure of deoxyribonucleic acid (DNA), the molecule that contains the genetic information of nearly all living organisms. Few discoveries have matched theirs in the understanding of the makeup of the human species. This discovery led to the 1990 founding of the Human Genome Project, a U.S.-initiated and funded undertaking through the Department of Energy and the National Institutes of Health and in collaboration with geneticists from China, France, Germany, Japan and the United Kingdom. Its goal was to code three billion nucleotides contained in the human genome and to identify all the genes present in it. This dramatic undertaking has given us a greater grasp of many of life's most basic—and traumatic—questions.

The Project's efforts have led to the discovery of approximately 35,000 genes.

Twenty percent of these genes have already been patented. Put another way, one-fifth of the blueprint that makes you . . .

me . . . our children . . . all of us . . . who we are is owned by someone else. And we have absolutely no say in what those patent holders do with our genes.

This cannot be what Watson and Crick intended.

The Dangers of Gene Patenting

Here are a few examples of the implications of gene patenting:

1. Gene patents interfere with research on diagnoses and cures. Half of all laboratories have stopped developing diagnostic tests because of concerns about infringing gene patents. One laboratory in four has had to abandon a clinical test in progress because of gene patents.

2. In countries where genes are not patented patients get better tests for genetic diseases than in the United States.

3. Forty-seven percent of geneticists have been denied requests from other faculty members for information, data, or materials regarding published research. The practice of withholding data detrimentally affects the training of the next generation of scientists. Almost one fourth of doctoral students and postdoctoral fellows reported they have been denied access to information, data and materials.

4. Disease-causing bacteria and viruses have now been patented. The genome of the virus that causes Hepatitis C, for example, is owned. This can lead to major problems, for if someone else wants to introduce inexpensive, timely public health testing for this (or another) common infectious disease, the patent holder can prevent it.

5. Few in this chamber would ever forget the SARS epidemic. From November 2002 to July 2003, this respiratory disease spread to 24 countries, killing 774 of the 8,096 people who contracted it. Scientists were apprehensive about vigorously studying the disease because

three patent applications were pending and they were fearful of possibly facing charges of patent infringement and subsequent litigation.

This is a serious problem and it is growing.

Fix the Mistake

My legislation, the Genomic Research and Accessibility Act, is straightforward: it ends the practice of gene patenting. It gives guidance to the United States Patent and Trademark Office (PTO) on what is not patentable—in this case, genetic material, naturally-occurring or modified. It is not retroactive—it does not rescind the patents already issued. But, fortunately, the Framers of our Constitution in their infinite wisdom made the point that any recognized invention deserved a monopoly for only a limited time. Congress has defined that scope of protected status to be 20 years from the point the patent application was filed. Thus, if we enact this bill into law quickly, we will reach balance in less than two decades—a patent-free genome that does not hinder scientific research, business enterprise, or human morality.

I do not wish to lay blame on anyone who has sought out a gene patent, for they all saw an opportunity and capitalized on it. But that opportunity should never have existed in the first place, and thus, it is time that we as a legislative body put an end to this practice.

Nor do I find fault with the Patent and Trademark Office. These days, it should not surprise anyone that innovative technology often outpaces innovative policies. Quite frankly, I don't know if the Patent and Trademark Office or anyone else for that matter had the technical expertise to fully understand the implications when the PTO granted the first gene patents. Those first patents set the precedent. The precedent created the practice. And the practice has now proliferated. This would not be the first time in our nation's history where government

Patent Law Unsuitable for Genes

A major part of the problem [with gene patenting] stems from the transfer of patent law from the sphere of chemistry and physics to the living world. In connection with chemistry, so-called product patents can be granted. These cover all properties of the patented substances, independently of whether they are described in the patent specification or not. Only *one single* commercial application needs to be stated in order to receive exclusive control of the substance and *all* its properties. This model was transferred to the genetic code. If one commercial application is described, the patent protects all biological functions of the gene inasmuch as they can be commercially exploited.

Now that the human genome has been decoded and it has become evident that genes usually perform several and often very different functions, this type of patent appears completely inappropriate. Genes now appear to be much more like encoded information than like active chemical substances. The genes that govern the laying of eggs in the threadworm may be responsible for Alzheimer's in human beings. Genes that cause breast cancer may also play an important role in diseases of the colon or prostate gland. . . .

An additional factor is that, unlike with chemical substances, it is rarely possible to circumvent a patent on genetic information by inventing a new chemical substance, particularly because the number of human genes is finite. Once these have been analyzed and patented, the blockade effect is much more extensive than in the case of chemical substances, whose number can be constantly increased by means of variations and experimental modifications.

Greenpeace, The True Cost of Gene Patents, *March 2004.*

has had to play catch up in order to properly understand technological innovation, and it certainly won't be the last.

Precedent does not and should not simply guarantee continued practice. Indeed, Congress has the constitutional right to proliferate and reward the advancement of invention, but it also has the responsibility to intervene should that advancement be misdirected or incorrect. Article I, Section 8 of the United States Constitution states that we must "promote the progress of science and useful arts, by securing for limited times to authors and inventors the exclusive right to their respective writings and discoveries." But implicit in those words is the power of discretion—Congress' charge to offer guidance on what exactly merits an exclusive right.

Genes Are Products of Nature

I make the argument that the human genome was not created by man, but instead is the very blueprint that creates man. The genome and the approximately 35,000 genes it encompasses has existed for millions of years, predating the human species; and suffice to say that it will certainly postdate us as well.

If you agree with me that genes have existed beyond the full grasp of human knowledge and indeed before the dawn of humankind, then you must conclude as I have that they are a product of nature and thus not patentable. Patenting the gene for breast cancer or any other gene is the analogous equivalent to patenting water, air, birds or diamonds.

But don't take my word for it. . . . One need only read the Supreme Court's *Diamond v. Chakrabarty* decision of 1980 to receive guidance on what is truly not patentable. In this landmark decision, Chief Justice William Burger wrote that "The laws of nature, physical phenomena, and abstract ideas have been held not patentable. . . . Thus, a new mineral discovered in the earth or a new plant found in the wild is not patentable subject matter. Likewise, Einstein could not patent his celebrated law that E=mc²; nor could Newton have patented the law of gravity. Such discoveries are [as the Constitution states,] 'manifestations of . . . nature, free to all men and reserved exclusively to none.'"

Proponents of gene patenting have said they are not patenting genes but instead are patenting "isolated and purified" genetic sequences. This is mere wordplay. In practice, these patents are patents on products of nature. For example, a patent on the supposedly isolated and purified breast cancer sequence prohibits a woman's doctor from looking for the breast cancer gene in her blood without paying $3,000 to the patent holder. It prohibits the same woman from donating her breast cancer gene to other researchers because the holder of the patent has the exclusive right to prevent anyone else from doing research on any individual's breast cancer gene. Such restrictions make clear that in effect, patents on isolated and purified sequences are patents on the actual genes found in nature.

Encouraging Further Scientific Advancement

We have overstepped our bounds. We have made a regulatory mistake. We have allowed the patenting of a product of nature.

Fortunately, we have the power to end the practice expeditiously and for the benefit of all. This bill will allow all doctors and researchers to have access to the genetic sequence, consisting of the chemical letters A (adenine), T (thymine), C (cytosine) and G (guanine). Just as we would never allow a patent on the alphabet that would permit the patent holder to charge people a royalty every time they spoke, we should not allow a patent on the genetic alphabet that comprises our common genome. . . .

Enacting the Genomic Research and Accessibility Act does not hamper invention, indeed, it encourages it. Medical innovation and economic advancement will occur if the study of genes is allowed to happen unabated. Incredible manifestations of intellectual property will result: medicines, machines, processes—most deserving of recognition, some potentially life-saving, and all worthy of a patent.

> "All food packages should be unmistak-
> ably labeled so we can make informed
> decisions about what we put into our
> bodies."

Genetically Modified Foods Should Be Labeled

Megan Tady

In the following viewpoint, Megan Tady asserts that many foods approved by the U.S. Food and Drug Administration contain genetically modified elements and other unspecified components. Tady argues that these foods should clearly be labeled so that consumers know when they are purchasing modified products. Tady maintains it is the consumer's right to know what goes into store-bought foods. Megan Tady is a national political reporter for In These Times, *a national magazine of political commentary.*

As you read, consider the following questions:

1. What two government agencies does the author fault for not enforcing labeling measures?

Megan Tady, "Recipe for Disaster: What's (Not) in a Food Label?" *In These Times*, October 4, 2007. Reproduced by permission of the publisher, www.inthesetimes.com.

2. What term did the Food and Drug Administration propose should replace that of *irradiation* on irradiated meat products, according to Tady?

3. According to a May 2007 poll cited by the author, what percentage of American consumers want cloned food to be labeled?

A decade after high school, and I'm still being served mystery meat.

Oh sure, a label is slapped onto the package, but the secret isn't in the calorie count. The unaccounted for ingredients—or rather, what's been done to my food before it becomes dinner—is being quietly and covertly left off of the label.

Hungry? No, I could go for an antacid. The realization that the public is left entirely in the dark about what's going in the pan really churns my stomach.

Refusing to Label "Frankenfoods"

It's the federal Food and Drug Administration (FDA) and the Department of Agriculture (USDA) that are the lunch ladies who won't share the recipe. Fortunately, the recipe isn't too difficult to find:

One part cloned meat: [In September 2007, the California legislature passed the first law mandating labels that disclose cloned meat or dairy products. The bill is now marinating on Governor [Arnold] Schwarzenegger's desk. As for the rest of us, we may be stuck eating Dolly [the first cloned sheep]. In 2006, the FDA announced that cloned meat and dairy products are safe for human consumption, and may market the food without any label identifying how it was made.

One part genetically modified (GM) food: Just because your box of cornflakes is void of a GM notice doesn't mean it's not a frankenfood. The FDA refuses to label food that has been genetically modified, so consumers have no clue when they're ingesting something that's been altered. What's more, the FDA may not even know which food contains GM ingredients; the agency only requires companies developing GM food to voluntarily submit to an evaluation process.

One part "organic" seafood: The USDA has yet to set any organic standards for seafood. Odd, then, that "organic" seafood is popping up in the freezer section. What's disturbing is that the USDA is allowing imported seafood to be labeled organic despite the absence of a standard.

One part food of unknown origin: With recent news of food contamination in everything from spinach to peanut butter to toothpaste, carefully selecting what we purchase has become essential. But with the [George W.] Bush administration continually delaying country-of-origin labeling on food, we still can't avoid products from places with dubious safety records.

And, finally, one part irradiated meat: Currently, consumers can see when they're purchasing meat that has been irradiated—a practice used to ward off contamination—thanks to a disclosure on the package. In April [2007], however, the FDA proposed a plan to yank this label and allow industry to replace the eerie term "irradiation" with the more palatable "pasteurization." And along with the word play, the FDA is considering removing the requirement for any label on any radiation that doesn't cause "material change" to the meat.

Consumers Cannot Decide for Themselves

Whether consumers should even be offered cloned, irradiated and GM food is for another dinnertime discussion. What's immediately troubling is that without labels and full disclosure, we can't decide for ourselves whether we want to be eating this food.

If you're put off by Today's Special, you're not the only one. Several consumer rights groups have been petitioning the FDA and USDA to halt this blind taste test and begin adequately labeling food.

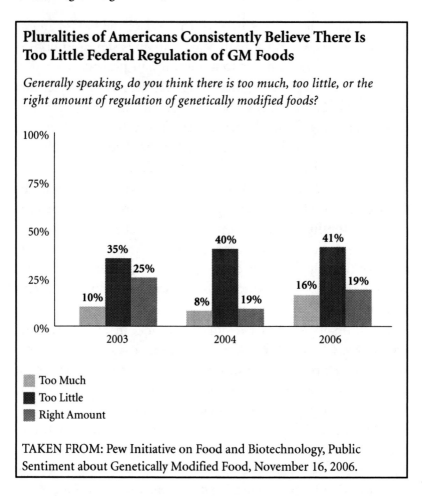

Pluralities of Americans Consistently Believe There Is Too Little Federal Regulation of GM Foods

Generally speaking, do you think there is too much, too little, or the right amount of regulation of genetically modified foods?

- Too Much
- Too Little
- Right Amount

TAKEN FROM: Pew Initiative on Food and Biotechnology, Public Sentiment about Genetically Modified Food, November 16, 2006.

Rebecca Spector, West Coast director for the Center for Food Safety, likened the absence of food labeling to an uncontrolled human experiment. "The public is really the guinea pigs in terms of safety issues," she says.

Controversy abounds about the safety of cloned meat and GM food, which industry and the government maintain are healthy for human consumption. But as Spector says, "The problem is, without labels, we have no way of tracing if there are adverse reactions. The industry will say, 'We have no evidence of adverse effects to genetically-engineered foods.' Well how would we know because we can't trace it back?"

It isn't that the government is fulfilling a consumer demand for ignorance. Poll after poll shows that we want to know what's on our forks. A May 2007 survey by Consumers Union found that 89 percent of Americans want labels on cloned food. In July [2007], the Consumers Union released a survey that found that 91 percent of the 1,000 people polled thought seafood labeled "organic" should reflect fish that is either free [of] or low in mercury and PCBs [polychlorinated biphenyls; compounds commonly used in pesticides]. Shame that the only thing accurate about the current label of "organic" seafood is the spelling.

More Cost than Benefit?

Knowing what's in our food and having the power to choose what we eat seems like a basic right. So why, like parents who think they know what's best for a child, is the FDA and USDA keeping this vital and fundamental information from us?

The FDA did not respond to an interview request, but Spector was quick to answer, saying food labels are a "regulatory burden" for the government and for industry, which routinely opposes disclosure. This reasoning is made clear on a USDA web page about country-of-origin labeling: "Mandatory labels are unlikely to increase food demand and likely will generate more costs than benefits." Treating our health as if it's a commodity, our government is privileging profit over consumer choice.

I'll be as clear as the government should be: All food packages should be unmistakably labeled so we can make informed decisions about what we put into our bodies. Until then, hand me another antacid and close the menu. Looks like dinner's already been decided for me.

| "What consumers have 'the right to know' is that mandatory labels for GM food would . . . add to shoppers' confusion, as well as to their grocery bills."

Genetically Modified Foods Should Not Be Labeled

Eli Kintisch

In the following viewpoint, Washington, D.C.–based reporter Eli Kintisch claims that labeling genetically engineered foods or foods that contain genetically modified (GM) components would be impractical. Kintisch argues that most foods contain traces of GM products, and therefore too many foods would be subject to labeling. The cost of this enterprise and the regulatory bureaucracy involved would be staggering, Kintisch adds. Thus, he suggests that those producers that want to market GM-free foods should label their products instead.

As you read, consider the following questions:

1. Why does Kintisch say that labeling of products containing more than 1 percent GM parts would not be a successful compromise in America?

2. According to the author, what would be the only way to ensure that manufacturers' ingredients do not come from GM sources?

3. Why does Kintisch believe that GM products will likely sell better than their non-GM counterparts?

"Americans have consistently demanded the right to know what's in their food," Senator Barbara Boxer righteously informed participants in a hearing on the labeling of genetically modified (GM) food [in] September [2000]. "[W]hy not tell Americans whether the ingredients in their food are natural or genetically engineered?" It's a popular plea. During the [2000] presidential campaign, both [Democratic candidate] Al Gore and [independent candidate] Ralph Nader promised mandatory labels on GM food. According to a Harris poll, 86 percent of Americans support the idea. "It's the very least that food producers can do," explains Craig Culp of Greenpeace. "People should be able to make informed decisions about what they eat." The argument is simple, commonsensical— and wrong. What consumers have "the right to know" is that mandatory labels for GM food would, in all likelihood, add to shoppers' confusion, as well as to their grocery bills.

Too Many to Label

When people talk about labeling GM food, they're generally thinking of the vegetable aisle of the supermarket. And if labeling simply meant putting a sticker on the genetically modified tomatoes of the future, it would make sense. But pumped-up fruits and vegetables are just the tip of the GM iceberg. Genetically engineered components—oil from GM soybeans, sugar from GM beets, flour from GM corn—also show up in lots of processed food. In fact, according to Greenpeace, they're present in more than 60 percent of the items on grocery-store shelves. (And, needless to say, they've caused no known health problems at all.) So do you slap labels on these products too? Keep in mind that while the oils, sugars, and flours in question come from genetically modified plants, the ingredients themselves usually are chemically indistinguishable from their non-GM equivalents. Complicating the issue still further are foods—such as beer, yogurt, bread, and cheese—that contain no GM ingredients at all but may be processed by genetically customized enzymes and microorganisms. Should we label these as well?

Given the quiet ubiquity of GM ingredients and processing in the food we already eat, a catchall GM label would be too broad to provide consumers with much guidance. In England, where food manufacturers began voluntarily labeling products containing GM ingredients in 1997, Jackie Dowthwaite of Britain's Food and Drink Federation says that "roughly half of the products in the supermarkets had the labels." And, just to be safe, many manufacturers labeled products as GM even if they weren't sure whether the sugar or flour or oil in them came from GM plants—thus making it impossible for consumers to make informed decisions.

Alternatively, you could label only products that contain GM substances in reasonably large doses—say, 1 percent of the combined ingredients. (This is, in fact, the standard that the 15 European Union countries—including Britain—adopted [in] January [2000].) But this compromise doesn't really address the concerns that prompted the labeling movement in the first place. For activists morally opposed to "meddling" with nature, a 1 percent meddling threshold is still unacceptable. And for those truly concerned about the safety of GM food, it's not much of a safeguard. "We worry about toxic substances in foods that appear at a level of 0.00001 percent," says Joseph Hotchkiss, a professor of food science and toxicology at Cornell University.

More Regulation, More Bureaucracy

What's more, even if labeling were required only for food modified beyond some arbitrary threshold, you'd still have the

Labeling Confusion

Terms like "not genetically modified" and "GMO [genetically modified organism] free," that include the word "modified" are not technically accurate unless they are clearly in a context that refers to bioengineering technology. "Genetic modification" means the alteration of the genotype of a plant using any technique, new or traditional. "Modification" has a broad context that means the alteration in the composition of food that results from adding, deleting, or changing hereditary traits, irrespective of the method. Modifications may be minor, such as a single mutation that affects one gene, or major alterations of genetic material that affect many genes. Most, if not all, cultivated food crops have been genetically modified. Data indicate that consumers do not have a good understanding that essentially all food crops have been genetically modified and that bioengineering technology is only one of a number of technologies used to genetically modify crops. Thus, while it is accurate to say that a bioengineered food was "genetically modified," it likely would be inaccurate to state that a food that had not been produced using biotechnology was "not genetically modified" without clearly providing a context so that the consumer can understand that the statement applies to bioengineering.

U.S. Food and Drug Administration, January 17, 2001.

problem of manufacturers who have no idea how much GM food—if any—their products contain. As in Britain, an American manufacturer of breakfast cereal, for example, may not know where the sugars and oils in its granola come from. Commercial crops such as corn and soybeans are sold in vast quantities, with GM and non-GM plants often inadvertently mixed together. When these crops are processed into oil and other products, things become more confusing still. By the time those products reach the granola manufacturer, there's no telling whether they contain some GM substances or not. After all, soybean and corn oils extracted from GM plants are chemically identical to those from non-GM ones.

The only way to ensure that a given ingredient comes from non-GM sources would be to create separate production lines from field to factory to grocery store. This wouldn't just require additional paperwork and regulatory bureaucracy to keep the GM and non-GM streams segregated. It would require entirely new grain bins, trucks, and cleaning procedures to ensure that non-GM crops and products were not "contaminated" by GM varieties as they were harvested, stored, shipped, and processed. Joe Parcell, an economist at the University of Missouri, estimates that segregating GM and non-GM soybeans could add "up to a dollar of segregation costs" to a $5 to $6 bushel of soybeans. A study for the Canadian market by KPMG Consulting projects that such segregation would force a recall-price markup of as much as 10 percent for food containing corn, canola, and soy-based products. For crops such as corn, whose GM varieties can transmit their genes to plants in adjacent fields via pollen, the costs of segregation could be even higher. The Chicago Federal Reserve warned that, in addition to raising prices at the supermarket, the burden of segregating GM and non-GM crops could make "smaller and higher-cost [agriculture] firms less viable." And this burden will only grow as the food industry uses greater and greater varieties of GM ingredients.

Anti-GM activists claim that in the 1990s the food industry used a similar cost "myth" to try to avoid the standardized "Nutrition Facts" labels now on foods. But Cornell's Hotchkiss argues that GM labeling will cost "a lot more." Moreover, the cost will be borne by consumers generally, whether or not they want to avoid GM-labeled food. "The major expense is not putting the label on," says University of Saskatchewan research scientist Alan McHughen, "it's keeping it off."

Label Non-GM Foods

All of which points to a solution that would help consumers make informed choices, limit the confusion caused by ubiquitous labels, and raise prices only for those consumers who consider GM food a problem: voluntary, standardized labeling of food *without* GM ingredients. Only companies that wanted to label their products "GM-free" would have to pay for the attendant segregation, quality control, and verification—and they would pass those costs along to their customers. Toward this end, the Food and Drug Administration, which rejected mandatory labeling [in May 2000], is already drafting guidelines that define when manufacturers can use a "non-GM" label. And the U.S. Department of Agriculture announced that food labeled "organic" would not contain GM ingredients, giving consumers an additional way to choose.

A "non-GM" label has the virtue of recognizing that GM-free products are now the exception at your local supermarket, rather than the rule. Consumers willing to pay the extra cost for such specialty products would be able to do so—just as millions of Americans already buy food certified kosher or organic. Those unconcerned about genetic tinkering wouldn't have to fund an extensive labeling regime. And the market would take it from there. If, as anti-GM activists argue, a majority of shoppers would pay extra to avoid GM food, we'd find out. Fueled by consumer demand, the GM-free niche would expand until it began pushing GM food off the shelves. On the other hand, if Americans generally prefer the cost, taste, or whatever of the bioengineered food they've been eating unknowingly (and without ill effect) for years, they'd have that option as well. And evidence suggests that many would take it. Even in the midst of Britain's political firestorm over GM food, tomato paste clearly labeled PRODUCED FROM GENETI-

CALLY MODIFIED TOMATOES sold better than its non-GM competitor in Sainsbury's supermarkets, a British chain. Why? The GM variety, says a company representative, was cheaper.

Periodical Bibliography

The following articles have been selected to supplement the diverse views presented in this chapter.

Current Events	"Has Genetic Engineering Gone Too Far?" April 16, 2007.
Economist	"Patent Pending," June 16, 2007.
Bernadine Healy	"Threats to Your Genetic Privacy," *U.S. News & World Report*, November 26, 2007.
Kyle Jensen and Fiona Murray	"Intellectual Property Landscape of the Human Genome," *Science*, October 14, 2005.
Jon F. Merz and Mildred K. Cho	"What Are Gene Patents and Why Are People Worried About Them?" *Community Genetics*, vol. 8, 2005.
Andrew Pollack	"Justices Drop Consideration of Boundaries for Patents," *New York Times*, June 23, 2006.
Brian Roe and Mario F. Teisl	"Genetically Modified Food Labeling: The Impacts of Message and Messenger on Consumer Perceptions of Labels and Products," *Food Policy*, February 2007.
Scientific American	"Private, Historical and Genetic Truths," July 2008.
Kara Sissell	"Lawsuit Seeks Mandatory Testing and Labeling of Genetically Modified Foods," *Chemical Week*, June 14, 2006.
Jeffrey M. Smith	"Protect Yourself from Genetically Modified Foods," *Total Health*, August 2005.
Gary Stix	"Owning the Stuff of Life," *Scientific American*, February 2006.
Rebecca Vesely	"Breaking the Code," *Modern Healthcare*, May 12, 2008.

For Further Discussion

Chapter 1

1. Nick Bostrom argues that human genetic enhancement is a natural extension of human inquiry into the unknown as well as a reflection of humanity's desire to improve itself. Like most transhumanist thinkers, Bostrom sees genetic manipulation as a means to overcome human shortcomings and reach beyond current limitations. How do you feel about Bostrom's arguments? Do they seem a natural outgrowth of human history; that is, given the way humanity has used technology in the past, do you believe that people would use genetic engineering to reach new states of consciousness and experience? Defend your answer.

2. Hugh McLachlan maintains that cloned humans should not be feared because they will be individuals who are different in most respects from their gene donors. Wendy Wright, however, contends that cloning humans would create a society in which individuals are devalued because they are merely genetic material waiting to be copied. After reading the viewpoints by McLachlan and Wright, explain whether you believe cloning is a dangerous science that ought to be avoided or is a technology that can improve human life.

3. Former U.S. senator Bill Frist supports government funding of embryonic stem cell research because he believes using embryos that are only going to be destroyed anyway is worthwhile if it leads to cures for diseases that are devastating to humankind and will continue to be so if unchecked. Do you agree with Frist's view? After reading President George W. Bush's viewpoint on stem cell re-

search, explain whether you think it is morally acceptable to tamper with any embryonic stem cells in the search for cures.

Chapter 2

1. What ethical objections does Michael J. Sandel have against human genetic enhancement? How does David Koepsell challenge ethical arguments against genetic engineering? After defining both ethical views, select the opinion you find more ethically sound and explain why you support it.

2. What are Britt Bailey's chief ethical objections to genetically modified (GM) food? Do you believe, like Bailey, that these concerns should halt the production of GM crops and livestock? If not, what ethical reasons are there to continue the manufacture and distribution of GM foods?

Chapter 3

1. Karri Hammerstrom contends that genetically modified crops are both environmentally safe and present no risk to humans when consumed. In her viewpoint, she begins by informing the reader that she is a mother and a consumer and later goes on to state that she is also a farmer. Why does she do this and how does it affect her argument? Do you trust her more because of her background? Why or why not? Weigh these feelings against those that you have when reading the viewpoint authored by the Union for Concerned Scientists, which maintains that genetically engineered crops present many potential risks for both human health and the environment. What is the background of the author in this case, and how does it impact your agreement with or skepticism of the viewpoint? Finally, which argument is most compelling? Explain your answer.

2. Many who argue for the continued use and development of genetically modified (GM) foods and crops tout the ways in which these crops could potentially alleviate hunger worldwide. Still others contend that implementing programs that focus on providing GM crops to impoverished people ignores the larger issues that cause hunger, making these programs, at best, only a temporary fix. Conduct further research to find out what, if any, consensus exists as to the causes of hunger. Based on your findings, do you believe, as stated by Gregory Conko and C.S. Prakash, that GM crops could be a solution to world hunger? Or do you agree with Carl F. Jordan, who states that policies involving GM crops only distract attention from the larger problems causing hunger? Or would a solution to world hunger include both the use of GM crops and attention to the larger social and economic problems that plague impoverished nations? Use evidence from your research and the viewpoints to support you view.

3. In stating that cloned animals should not be used for food, Joseph Mendelson III makes his argument by focusing on two major issues: the safety risks to humans who eat clone-derived food and the welfare of animals. If cloned animals are deemed safe for consumption, how important is the issue of animal welfare to your decision about whether clones should be used in food production? Siobhan DeLancey, Larisa Rudenko, and John Matheson explain the benefits, for both farmers and consumers, of using cloned animals for food. Do you believe that these benefits outweigh the costs outlined by Mendelson? If cloning produces a product superior to what can be achieved through traditional breeding methods, would animal welfare issues be sufficient reason to ban cloning in food production? Explain your answer.

Chapter 4

1. Gene patents have raised questions about who should be allowed to "own" and profit from discoveries relating to the genetic building blocks of life. Geoffrey M. Karny and others who support human gene patents argue that without these patents, the incentive for and ability to conduct genetic research would disappear, and as a result scientific discovery in the field of genetics would be reduced. Xavier Becerra and others who oppose the patenting of human genes maintain that gene patents only make it more difficult for those who want to conduct research, due to royalty payments and possible litigation connected with patents. After reviewing each viewpoint, which argument do you find more convincing? Explain why.

2. Eli Kintisch claims that labeling genetically modified food would be impractical because of the bureaucracy it would create and the difficulty involved in labeling every food item that contains even trace amounts of GM products. Other detractors of labeling have argued that labeling would scare consumers who normally buy products with some amount of GM food content. Do you support either of these views, or do believe that labeling of GM products should be mandatory and can be practical? Explain your answer.

Organizations to Contact

The editors have compiled the following list of organizations concerned with the issues debated in this book. The descriptions are derived from materials provided by the organizations. All have publications or information available for interested readers. The list was compiled on the date of publication of the present volume; the information provided here may change. Be aware that many organizations take several weeks or longer to respond to inquiries, so allow as much time as possible.

Center for Bioethics and Human Dignity (CBHD)
2065 Half Day Rd., Deerfield, IL   60015
(847) 317-8180 • fax: (847) 317-8101
e-mail: info@cbhd.org
Web site: www.cbhd.org

CBHD examines the issues of bioethics using rigorous research and analytical techniques while also taking into account biblical values and their influence on Western culture and ethics. The organization opposes cloning and stem cell research that destroys human embryos. Additional topics addressed by the organization include biotechnology, genetics, and reproductive ethics. Articles concerning these issues and others can be found online, and the CBHD Web site also posts audio files and transcripts of the *Bioethics Podcast*, where experts discuss bioethics in contemporary society.

Center for Food Safety (CFS)
660 Pennsylvania Ave. SE, #302, Washington, DC   20003
(202) 547-9359 • fax: (202) 547-9429
e-mail: office@centerforfoodsafety.org
Web site: www.centerforfoodsafety.org

CFS was founded by the International Center for Technology Assessment in 1997 to assess new technologies being used for food production and to offer alternative methods that provide sustainable food sources. The organization provides educational materials to the public and the media, and suggests guidelines to policy makers. CFS opposes the commercial release of genetically engineered food products without rigorous testing to ensure their safety, contends that all genetically engineered foods should be labeled, and believes that cloned animals should not be used in food production. Reports on these topics and others can be read on the CFS Web site.

Council for Responsible Genetics (CRG)
5 Upland Rd., Suite 3, Cambridge, MA   02140
(617) 868-0870 • fax: (617) 491-5344
e-mail: crg@gene-watch.org
Web site: www.gene-watch.org

CRG works to provide accurate and current information about emerging biotechnologies so that citizens can play a more active role in shaping policies regarding these advances. Specific topics addressed by the organization include genetic determinism, cloning and human genetic manipulation, and constructing and promoting a "Genetic Bill of Rights." *Gene Watch* is the bimonthly publication of CRG; articles from this magazine as well as other institute reports are accessible on the CRG Web site.

Greenpeace
702 H St. NW, Suite 300, Washington, DC   20001
(202) 462-1177
e-mail: info@wdc.greenpeace.org
Web site: www.greenpeace.org

Greenpeace is an activist group seeking to protect the environment worldwide. Current interests of the organization include combating global warming, deforestation, and ocean pollution. Additionally, Greenpeace opposes the genetic engineering (GE) of food and food sources, and contends that any GE food on the market should be labeled. Reports on the threat of genetic engineering to the environment, as well as reports on other topics can be downloaded from the Greenpeace Web site.

Institute on Biotechnology and the Human Future (IBHF)

565 W. Adams St., Chicago, IL   60661
(312) 906-5377
e-mail: info@thehumanfuture.org
Web site: www.thehumanfuture.org

IBHF examines the research on current and emerging biotechnologies and provides a forum for discussion between individuals of all backgrounds on the cultural significance and ethical issues surrounding these technologies, with the ultimate goal being the promotion of human life and progress. Areas of inquiry include genetic discrimination, gene patents, and human cloning. The IBHF Web site provides commentaries by experts on these topics and others.

International Bioethics Committee (IBC)

2 United Nations Plaza, Room 900, New York, NY   10017
(212) 963-5995 • fax: (212) 963-8014
e-mail: newyork@unesco.org
Web site: www.unesco.org/ibc

The IBC is a committee within the United Nations Educational, Scientific, and Cultural Organization. The thirty-six independent experts that make up the committee meet to ensure that human dignity and freedom are observed and respected in biotechnological advances worldwide. The IBC has authored declarations such as the *Universal Declaration on the Human Genome and Human Rights*, the *International Declaration on Human Genetic Data*, and the *Universal Declaration on Bioethics and Human Rights*, to provide guidelines for those working in the fields of biotechnology. These declarations, as well as other publications, can be viewed online at the organization's Web site.

International Center for Technology Assessment (ICTA)

660 Pennsylvania Ave. SE, Suite 302, Washington, DC   20003
(202) 547-9359 • fax: (202) 547-9429
e-mail: info@icta.org
Web site: www.icta.org

ICTA works to educate the public about the economic, social, environmental, and political impacts of technology on society. The center opposes the patenting of genes and seeks to promote legislation to regulate human biotechnology to ensure its ethical use. The ICTA Web site provides reports on patents, human biotechnology, and other topics.

National Human Genome Research Institute (NHGRI)
National Institutes of Health, Bldg. 31, Room 4B09
9000 Rockville Pike, Bethesda, MD   20892-2152
(301) 402-0911 • fax: (301) 402-2218
Web site: www.genome.gov

NHGRI is a branch of the National Institutes of Health in the United States, established in 1989 to participate in the International Human Genome Project to map the human genome. Since the completion of the sequencing of the human genome, the institute has embarked on the mission of further researching the genome to better understand how it functions in human health and disease. Additionally, NHGRI provides information about policy and ethics issues as well as educational material about human genetics. Detailed information about these and other topics can be searched and viewed on the NHGRI Web site.

Nuffield Council on Bioethics
Communications & External Affairs Manager
28 Bedford Square, London   WC1B 3JS
44 207 681 9619 • fax: 44 207 637 1712
e-mail: bioethics@nuffieldbioethics.org
Web site: www.nuffieldbioethics.org

Established in 1991, the Nuffield Council on Bioethics works to identify and address ethical issues connected with current and emerging biotechnologies. The council also provides educational information to the public to stimulate discussion and debate about these technologies. The Nuffield Council's Web site offers copies of papers it has published, such as *The Ethics of Patenting DNA*, *Genetically Modified Crops: Ethical and Social Issues*, and *Stem Cell Therapy: Ethical Issues*.

Sierra Club

85 Second St., 2nd Floor, San Francisco, CA   94105
(415) 977-5500 • fax: (415) 977-5799
e-mail: information@sierraclub.org
Web site: www.sierraclub.org

Founded in 1892, the Sierra Club works to ensure that the planet is protected and preserved. With regards to genetically engineered organisms (GEOs), Sierra Club maintains that a moratorium on the planting and release of any GEOs should be observed until extensive testing has been done to ensure their safety for both humans and the environment. The organization also opposes the patenting of GEOs and the genetic code of humans. *Sierra* is the bimonthly magazine of the Sierra Club; articles from this publication and others specific to the issue of genetic engineering are available online.

Union of Concerned Scientists (UCS)

2 Brattle Square, Cambridge, MA   02238-9105
(617) 547-5552 • fax: (617) 864-9405
Web site: www.ucsusa.org

UCS is a membership organization of citizens and scientists who work together to promote the responsible use of science to improve the world. UCS has extensively researched and reported on the use of genetic engineering (GE) in food and plant products, as well as on the cloning of animals in the food production chain, generally advocating a precautionary approach to the use of these products. The organization argues that more testing must be conducted before GE crops and cloned animals for food production can be considered safe and suitable for consumers. UCS publishes updates for those who subscribe to one of its email lists. The UCS Web site provides additional reports and fact sheets.

U.S. Food and Drug Administration (FDA)

5600 Fishers Ln., Rockville, MD   20857-0001
(888) 463-6332
Web site: www.fda.gov

The FDA is the U.S. government agency responsible for ensuring the quality and safety of all food and drug products sold in the United States. As such, the FDA has conducted extensive tests to evaluate the safety of genetically engineered (GE) foods and has issued guidelines and regulatory measures to control what types of GE products make it to market. The Center for Veterinary Medicine (CVM), an office within the FDA, specifically examines the impact of GE products on animals and has also researched and reported on the cloned animals that are used in the food industry. Reports by both the FDA and CVM can be retrieved from the FDA Web site.

Bibliography of Books

Nicholas Agar
Liberal Eugenics: In Defence of Human Enhancement. Malden, MA: Blackwell, 2004.

Michael Bellomo
The Stem Cell Divide: The Facts, the Fiction, and the Fear Driving the Greatest Scientific, Political, and Religious Debate of Our Time. New York: American Management Association, 2006.

Daniel Charles
Lords of the Harvest: Biotech, Big Money, and the Future of Food. Cambridge, MA: Perseus, 2001.

Nina V. Fedoroff and Nancy Marie Brown
Mendel in the Kitchen: A Scientist's View of Genetically Modified Foods. Washington, DC: Joseph Henry, 2004.

Francis Fukuyama
Our Posthuman Future: Consequences of the Biotechnology Revolution. New York: Farrar, Straus & Giroux, 2002.

Joel Garreau
Radical Evolution: The Promise and Peril of Enhancing Our Minds, Our Bodies—and What It Means to Be Human. New York: Doubleday, 2005.

Jonathan Glover
Choosing Children: Genes, Disability, and Design. New York: Oxford University Press, 2006.

Ronald M. Green
Babies by Design: The Ethics of Genetic Choice. New Haven, CT: Yale University Press, 2007.

John Harris — *Enhancing Evolution: The Ethical Case for Making Better People.* Princeton, NJ: Princeton University Press, 2007.

Eve Herold — *Stem Cell Wars: Inside Stories from the Frontlines.* New York: Palgrave Macmillan, 2006.

Leon R. Kass and James Q. Wilson — *The Ethics of Human Cloning.* Washington, DC: AEI Press, 1998.

Bill Lambrecht — *Dinner at the New Gene Café: How Genetic Engineering Is Changing What We Eat, How We Live, and the Global Politics of Food.* New York: Thomas Dunne, 2001.

Kerry Lynn Macintosh — *Illegal Beings: Human Clones and the Law.* New York: Cambridge University Press, 2005.

Barbara MacKinnon, ed. — *Human Cloning: Science, Ethics, and Public Policy.* Urbana: University of Illinois Press, 2000.

Jane Maienschein — *Whose View of Life? Embryos, Cloning, and Stem Cells.* Cambridge, MA: Harvard University Press, 2003.

Alan McHughen — *Pandora's Picnic Basket: The Potential and Hazards of Genetically Modified Foods.* New York: Oxford University Press, 2000.

Bill McKibben — *Enough: Staying Human in an Engineered Age.* New York: Times Books, 2003.

Ben C. Mitchell et al.	*Biotechnology and the Human Good.* Washington, DC: Georgetown University Press, 2007.
Ramez Naam	*More than Human: Embracing the Promise of Biological Enhancement.* New York: Broadway, 2005.
Robert Paarlberg	*Starved for Science: How Biotechnology Is Being Kept Out of Africa.* Cambridge, MA: Harvard University Press, 2008.
Gregory E. Pence	*Who's Afraid of Human Cloning?* Lanham, MD: Rowman & Littlefield, 1998.
Gregory E. Pence	Designer Food: Mutant Harvest or Breadbasket of the World? Lanham, MD: Rowman & Littlefield, 2002.
Peter Pringle	*Food, Inc.: Mendel to Monsanto—the Promises and Perils of the Biotech Harvest.* New York: Simon & Schuster, 2003.
Michael J. Sandel	*The Case Against Perfection: Ethics in the Age of Genetic Engineering.* Cambridge, MA: Belknap, 2007.
Jeffrey M. Smith	*Genetic Roulette: The Documented Health Risks of Genetically Engineered Foods.* White River Junction, VT: Chelsea Green, 2007.

Jeffrey M. Smith *Seeds of Deception: Exposing Industry and Government Lies About the Safety of the Genetically Engineered Foods You're Eating.* Fairfield, IA: Yes! Books, 2003.

Pam Solo and Gail Pressberg *The Promise and Politics of Stem Cell Research.* Westport, CT: Praeger, 2007.

Gregory Stock *Redesigning Humans: Our Inevitable Genetic Future.* Boston: Houghton Mifflin, 2002.

Martin Teitel and Kimberly A. Wilson *Genetically Engineered Food: Changing the Nature of Nature.* Rochester, VT: Park Street, 2001.

Brent Waters and Ronald Cole-Turner, eds. *God and the Embryo: Religious Voices on Stem Cells and Cloning.* Washington, DC: Georgetown University Press, 2003.

Paul Weirich, ed. *Labeling Genetically Modified Food: The Philosophical and Legal Debate.* New York: Oxford University Press, 2007.

Ian Wilmut and Roger Highfield *After Dolly: The Promise and Perils of Human Cloning.* New York: Norton, 2007.

Index